# The Fat-Free Truth

# The Fat-Free Truth

239 Real Answers to the
Fitness and Weight-Loss Questions
You Wonder About Most

Liz Neporent, M.A.,
and Suzanne Schlosberg

Houghton Mifflin Company
Boston • New York
2005

For information about permission to reproduce selections
from this book, write to Permissions, Houghton Mifflin Company,
215 Park Avenue South, New York, New York 10003.

Visit our Web site: www.houghtonmifflinbooks.com.

*Library of Congress Cataloging-in-Publication Data*
Neporent, Liz.
The fat-free truth : 239 real answers to the fitness and
weight-loss questions you wonder about most / Liz
Neporent and Suzanne Schlosberg.
p.  cm
Includes bibliographical references and index.
ISBN 0-618-31073-8
1. Weight loss  2. Physical fitness.  I. Schlosberg,
Suzanne.  II. Title.
RM222.2.N46 2005
613.7 — dc22    2004057682

ILLUSTRATIONS BY LAURA HARTMAN MAESTRO

BOOK DESIGN BY JOYCE C. WESTON

Printed in the United States of America

MP 10 9 8 7 6 5 4 3 2 1

This book includes information about a variety of topics related to diet,
exercise, and health. The ideas and suggestions contained in this book
are not intended as a substitute for the services of a trained professional
or the advice of a medical expert. The authors and publisher disclaim re-
sponsibility for any adverse effects resulting directly or indirectly from
information contained in this book.

# Contents

# Expert Reviewers

**Liz Applegate, Ph.D.**
Senior Lecturer, Department of Nutrition, University of California, Davis

**Cedric Bryant, Ph.D.**
Chief Physiologist, American Council on Exercise

**Paul Ernsberger, Ph.D.**
Associate Professor of Nutrition, Case Western Reserve School of Medicine

**Glenn Gaesser, Ph.D.**
Professor of Exercise Physiology
Director, Kinesiology Program, University of Virginia

**Scott Haltzman, M.D.**
Clinical Associate Professor, Department of Psychiatry and Human Behavior, Brown University
Medical Director, NRI Community Services, Woonsocket, Rhode Island

**Ralph LaForge, M.S.**
Exercise Physiologist, Duke University Medical Center

**John Martinez, P.T.**
Vice President of Physical Therapy, Plus One Health Management, New York, New York

**Joan Y. Meek, M.D., R.D.**
Director, General Academic Pediatrics, Orlando Regional Healthcare
Arnold Palmer Hospital for Children & Women

**Neal Pire, M.S.**
President, New York Regional Chapter, American College of Sports Medicine

# Acknowledgments

**From Liz and Suzanne:**

We're grateful to our editor, Susan Canavan, for her enthusiasm about this project and her guidance on the manuscript. We're also thankful to the following expert reviewers for their thorough evaluation and invaluable suggestions: Liz Applegate, Ph.D.; Cedric Bryant, Ph.D.; Paul Ernsberger, Ph.D.; Glenn Gaesser, Ph.D.; Scott Haltzman, M.D.; Ralph LaForge, M.S.; John Martinez, P.T.; Joan Y. Meek, M.D., R.D.; and Neal Pire, M.S.

**From Liz:**

I owe a debt of gratitude to Grace DeSimone, Neal Pire, Melissa McNeese, Etta Reyes, Rick Caro, Alex Ham, Diane Naiztat, and Stephen Harris for seeing me through the writing of this book as well as everything else that goes on in my life. The same goes to my wonderful agent, Linda Konner, and my favorite editor/sounding board, Mary Duffy. I'm also grateful to the entire American Council on Exercise for their support and to iVillage.com for giving me the opportunity to interact with women from all over the country who are as passionate about health and fitness as I am. I am indebted to my great friend Patty Buttenheim for, well, just about everything.

There is not a thank-you big enough to cover what Suzanne Schlosberg, my coauthor for nearly ten years, has done for me; she's taught me more about writing, research, and accuracy than anyone I've ever known.

Thanks to my parents; my brother Mark; his wife, Lisa; my sister, Jill; her husband, Ted; my brother Richard; and my cousins Margie Semilof and David Wildstein, for their love and encouragement. And finally, to my husband, Jay, whom I love more every day: I could not do any of this without you.

## From Suzanne:

This entire undertaking wouldn't have been possible without Nancy Gottesman, my *Shape* magazine Q&A editor for a decade. Perhaps she's not my most practical friend, but she's definitely the most patient: During the year it took to write this book, I was late turning in every single column. I am also immensely grateful to my "other Nancy," Nancy Kruh, for coming to my rescue with *The Curse of the Singles Table* so that I could focus on this book when I needed to. Speaking of rescues, I am also indebted to Richard Motzkin, my stellar agent.

Liz Neporent is a cabinet-level coauthor and friend; I'm constantly amazed at her wealth of knowledge and grateful for her excitement about the minutiae that make my eyes glaze over. My husband, Paul Spencer, was a great help on the research and technology fronts. Thanks also to Sarah Bowen Shea and Dana Sullivan for their help with the pregnancy questions and to Rita Burris for her emergency visit to the library.

All of my family members are incredibly supportive, but I would like to single out Grandpa Julius, who asked me virtually every single day for a year, "How's the book coming?" Gpa, you can buy your six copies now!

# The Fat-Free Truth

# Introduction

Have you heard?

> The Atkins diet has been vindicated by scientific research, and you can go ahead and eat pork chops to your heart's content.

> If you pack on 3 pounds of muscle, you'll burn an extra 10,000 calories a month.

> Pilates gives you "long, lean muscles — no bulk!"

> Pedaling backward on the elliptical machine tones your rear thighs better than peddling forward does.

You've probably heard all four of these statements at one time or another — from a TV news report, a newspaper article, a friend at your health club, or a fitness Web site. Each one sounds plausible, but how do you know if it's true?

That's the question that probably comes to mind with every new diet plan, metabolism-boosting pill, exercise device, and workout regimen you come across — and your own common sense tells you the promises can't all be true.

Indeed, there's no shortage of exaggerations and misconceptions floating around the media and the gym, and there's plenty of conflicting advice. That's why we've written this book. For more than a decade, the two of us have been answering fitness questions for national magazines, newspapers, and Web sites and, in Liz's case, at corporate gyms she has managed around the world. Every month, hundreds of readers and clients ask us for explanations, clarifications, and guidance on sorting through the barrage of contradictory information. "I'm totally confused!" they say. Or, "Help! I don't know which 'expert' to believe!" Often they're frustrated because they've invested time and money in one new regimen or another and failed to achieve the results they were promised.

Of course, it's no wonder the fitness-conscious public is befuddled. Every time a new study is published or report is issued, the conventional wisdom seems to get turned on its head. First we're told by an esteemed government panel that 30 minutes a day of exercise will suffice. But then another respected organization reports that we need 60 minutes. Whom to believe? On the one hand, we're told that working out at a slow pace burns more fat; on the other, we're told that exercising at a fast pace burns more calories. Which is the best approach?

Our goal is to give you straight-shooting answers to the workout and weight-loss questions that you wonder about most. Once you know what's fact and what's fiction — and, by the way, those first four statements are all, to varying degrees, fiction — you can confidently spend your time, effort, and money on strategies that actually work. You're sure to get better results if you base your fitness programs on the truth, not the hype or rumor.

We believe that an inquisitive nature is an essential part of a fitness or weight-loss program. Given the country's skyrocketing obesity rates and increasing demand for weight-loss plans and products, the market abounds with sneaky advertising tactics. It pays to be skeptical. But it also pays to keep your eyes and ears open for solid new research, programs, and gizmos that may represent genuine advances. While hucksters are polluting the airwaves and the Internet, scientists at respected universities are tackling exercise and diet issues that have long been ignored, offering insight into the pros and cons of popular eating plans, diet drugs, surgical procedures, fitness regimens, and exercise devices. Typically, this steady stream of fascinating research doesn't make it much farther than scientific journals, which aren't made easily accessible — or understandable — to the general public. Often, the research that does reach the public is misreported by the media. That's where this book comes in.

We've ignored the hype, scrutinized the studies, and quizzed the researchers, tackling commonly asked questions such as "How can I boost my metabolism?" and "What's the best way to get rid of a paunchy middle?" We've also addressed questions you might not even have thought of asking, including "What are my chances of regaining weight after liposuction?" and "Will I sweat more — or less — as I become more fit?" And just in case you find your-self stymied for conversation at a cocktail party, we've also tossed in some fitness trivia questions. Next time you need an ice-breaker, try this one out: "Say, does anyone know how the marathon came to be 26.2 miles?"

Not every question in this book has a definitive answer — but that's important for you to know, too. The people pushing the lat-est exercise or diet fad often make statements in black-and-white terms (you must eat this; you must never eat that), and media headlines aim for maximum impact in minimum space ("Atkins Works!" and "Eat Grapefruit, Shed Weight!"). But in reality, sci-ence moves at a slow pace, and many fitness and weight-loss con-troversies have yet to be sorted out. Often, the latest study is just one piece in a large puzzle that will take years, if not decades, to solve.

When there is a consensus on a topic, we let you know. When the answer to a question is simply unknown or unclear, we tell you that, too. In the absence of a rock-solid answer, the next best thing is perspective.

Many of the answers in this book are likely to surprise you. A number of them even surprised us, contradicting what we'd heard for years from trainers, nutritionists, and physicians. When we took a hard look at the published scientific studies, we found that, in some cases, the conventional wisdom didn't hold up. For ex-ample: We'd been told countless times that drinking water helps you lose weight by making you feel full. Turns out, that's not ex-actly what the research says.

In some cases, it wasn't the research that surprised us but the fact that we couldn't find any — or that it appeared to be more elusive than the Loch Ness monster. Consider the question, "Which burns more calories: the upright stationary bike or the recum-bent?" We started our research at the gym, where we found that the calorie readouts on both types of bikes came up identical. This made us suspicious; intuitively, we felt these activities are too dif-ferent to burn the exact same number of calories. So we cranked into investigation mode to find out: Is it true?

As it turned out, the "truth" was tough to track down. We scoured textbooks, surfed every wave on the Web, cross-examined everyone we knew with a Ph.D. attached to his or her name. Finally, we found a source who unearthed a pile of intriguing research at the University of Wisconsin library. From this we learned, as we explain in Question #135, that there is indeed a big difference between sitting upright as you pedal and reclining in a bucket seat.

Though some of the information presented in this book was a challenge to ferret out, we've made it easy for you to access. If there's a very specific topic you're interested in — such as yoga, weight-loss surgery, or treadmills — flip right to the index and you'll be directed to the relevant questions. If there's a more general subject you want to learn about — whether it's mind-body exercise, nutrition, or strength training — scan the table of contents and turn to the corresponding section. Within each part, related questions are grouped together. For the most succinct answer to any question — essentially, the sound bite — read the first paragraph of each answer, a.k.a. "the short answer." If you're intrigued, keep reading for a more thorough explanation, along with tips for putting the information into action.

As you read this book, odds are you'll find answers that make you go, "I knew it! I've been right all along!" as well as information that makes you think, "Hmm, maybe I'd better try a different approach." Whatever your reaction, you can be confident of one thing: You're getting the fat-free truth.

# Your Body:
# Fat, Weight, and Muscle

What's your dream weight? You probably have some number tucked away in your brain, and maybe you've started a program to achieve your goal. But how did you come up with that number? Is it what you weighed in college? Is it the weight of a certain celebrity you read about in *People* magazine? Is it the number you put on your driver's license because you think it's what you *should* weigh?

Most of us embark on weight-loss plans without considering one key question: Is my goal weight realistic for my body? Knowing the answer may save you a huge amount of frustration. This section explains the basics of body weight, body fat, and muscle, giving you the tools to set sensible weight goals and track your progress.

We also lay out the lingo about the human body that is commonly tossed around in media reports, at health clubs, and throughout this book — terms such as body mass index (BMI), body composition, and fast-twitch muscle fibers. We dispel some persistent myths about cellulite and fat cells and offer up compelling statistics about obesity rates over the years and around the world. Guess which nation is heftier: Greece or Japan? See Question #5 for the answer.

What this section boils down to: The more you know about your body, the more equipped you are to improve it.

## Question #1: How do I figure out my ideal weight?

*The short answer:* Actually, the whole concept of "ideal weight" isn't very useful, since the number on the scale doesn't tell you all that much about your health, your fitness, or even your svelteness. For better clues about whether you need to slim down, consider your body-fat percentage, body mass index, waist circumference, and health factors such as your blood pressure and cholesterol levels. Although each of these measures has its flaws, you can tell a lot about your weight (and health) by taking them all into consideration.

*You may have some weight* that in your mind triggers thoughts like, "Uh-oh, I'm getting fat!" or "Oh no, I'm headed for a heart attack." But assessing your plumpness or your risk for obesity-related diseases is not as simple as stepping on a scale. For one thing, your weight doesn't reveal how much of your body consists of fat (as opposed to, say, muscle, bones, blood, and organs). It's body fat — not total body weight — that plays a significant role in disease risk. A very rough way to estimate whether you have too much fat is to determine your body mass index, or BMI, explained in Question #2. A more precise way to gauge your body fat is to have it tested using any of the methods described in Question #8.

However, neither your BMI nor your body-fat percentage tells you anything about the location of your body fat — a more important indicator of disease risk than total fat. Fat in the abdominal region, clumped around your internal organs, poses a more serious threat than fat in your hips and thighs; in fact, research suggests, saddlebags may even offer some protection against cardiovascular disease. If you're a woman, a waist measurement over 35 inches puts you at greater health risk, according to the National Institutes of Health. For men, the critical number is 40 inches.

Finally, you need to consider other clues that may put your health at risk, including high blood pressure, high levels of LDL cholesterol (the "bad" cholesterol), low levels of HDL (the "good" cholesterol), high triglycerides (fat in your bloodstream), high blood-glucose levels, physical inactivity, a family history of premature heart disease, and cigarette smoking.

Your scale weight may give you a rough sense of whether

you're heading in a healthy or unhealthy direction, but it's important to consider the whole picture. If one measure is out of whack but the others are in the healthy range, you're probably okay. If several are on the high side, that's an indication you need to make some lifestyle changes. Your physician can help you put each measure in perspective and assess your risk for developing obesity-related diseases.

**Question #2: I've heard that my body mass index is more important than my weight. Why is this, and what is BMI, anyway?**

*The short answer:* Body mass index, or BMI, is a measure of your weight relative to your height — a rough gauge of how "fat" you are. A high BMI is one of several red flags for obesity-related diseases, but for many people, including athletes, BMI can be unreliable. Also, like scale weight, BMI doesn't tell you anything about how your fat is distributed, so it's of limited use.

*BMI isn't as well known* an acronym as FBI or IBM, but as the obesity epidemic has drawn more media attention, these three letters have entered the national vocabulary. Below are the BMI guidelines issued by the National Institutes of Health. Keep in mind that some experts consider these cutoffs to be arbitrary and emphasize that fitness may be more important than thinness when it comes to disease risk.

- BMI 18.5 or below: You're underweight.
- BMI between 18.5 and 24.9: You're in the healthy range.
- BMI between 25 and 29.9: You're overweight.
- BMI 30 or greater: You're obese.

If you consider your calculator a close personal friend and want to you know your precise BMI, use the following formula.

$$BMI = \frac{(\text{Weight in pounds})}{[(\text{Height in inches}) \times (\text{Height in inches})]} \times 703$$

## What's My Body Mass Index?

Locate your height in the left-hand column. Then move across until you find your weight. The number at the top of the column is your BMI. Pounds have been rounded off.

| BMI | 19 | 20 | 21 | 22 | 23 | 24 | 25 | 26 |
|---|---|---|---|---|---|---|---|---|
| Height (inches) | | | | Body Weight (pounds) | | | | |
| 58 | 91 | 96 | 100 | 105 | 110 | 115 | 119 | 124 |
| 59 | 94 | 99 | 104 | 109 | 114 | 119 | 124 | 128 |
| 60 | 97 | 102 | 107 | 112 | 118 | 123 | 128 | 133 |
| 61 | 100 | 106 | 111 | 116 | 122 | 127 | 132 | 137 |
| 62 | 104 | 109 | 115 | 120 | 126 | 131 | 136 | 142 |
| 63 | 107 | 113 | 118 | 124 | 130 | 135 | 141 | 146 |
| 64 | 110 | 116 | 122 | 128 | 134 | 140 | 145 | 151 |
| 65 | 114 | 120 | 126 | 132 | 138 | 144 | 150 | 156 |
| 66 | 118 | 124 | 130 | 136 | 142 | 148 | 155 | 161 |
| 67 | 121 | 127 | 134 | 140 | 146 | 153 | 159 | 166 |
| 68 | 125 | 131 | 138 | 144 | 151 | 158 | 164 | 171 |
| 69 | 128 | 135 | 142 | 149 | 155 | 162 | 169 | 176 |
| 70 | 132 | 139 | 146 | 153 | 160 | 167 | 174 | 181 |
| 71 | 136 | 143 | 150 | 157 | 165 | 172 | 179 | 186 |
| 72 | 140 | 147 | 154 | 162 | 169 | 177 | 184 | 191 |
| 73 | 144 | 151 | 159 | 166 | 174 | 182 | 189 | 197 |
| 74 | 148 | 155 | 163 | 171 | 179 | 186 | 194 | 202 |
| 75 | 152 | 160 | 168 | 176 | 184 | 192 | 200 | 208 |
| 76 | 156 | 164 | 172 | 180 | 189 | 197 | 205 | 213 |

| 27 | 28 | 29 | 30 | 31 | 32 | 33 | 34 | 35 | 36 |
|----|----|----|----|----|----|----|----|----|----|
| | | | **Body Weight (pounds)** | | | | | | |
| 129 | 134 | 138 | 143 | 148 | 153 | 158 | 162 | 167 | 172 |
| 133 | 138 | 143 | 148 | 153 | 158 | 163 | 168 | 173 | 178 |
| 138 | 143 | 148 | 153 | 158 | 163 | 168 | 174 | 179 | 184 |
| 143 | 148 | 153 | 158 | 164 | 169 | 174 | 180 | 185 | 190 |
| 147 | 153 | 158 | 164 | 169 | 175 | 180 | 186 | 191 | 196 |
| 152 | 158 | 163 | 169 | 175 | 180 | 186 | 191 | 197 | 203 |
| 157 | 163 | 169 | 174 | 180 | 186 | 192 | 197 | 204 | 209 |
| 162 | 168 | 174 | 180 | 186 | 192 | 198 | 204 | 210 | 216 |
| 167 | 173 | 179 | 186 | 192 | 198 | 204 | 210 | 216 | 223 |
| 172 | 178 | 185 | 191 | 198 | 204 | 211 | 217 | 223 | 230 |
| 177 | 184 | 190 | 197 | 203 | 210 | 216 | 223 | 230 | 236 |
| 182 | 189 | 196 | 203 | 209 | 216 | 223 | 230 | 236 | 243 |
| 188 | 195 | 202 | 209 | 216 | 222 | 229 | 236 | 243 | 250 |
| 193 | 200 | 208 | 215 | 222 | 229 | 236 | 243 | 250 | 257 |
| 199 | 206 | 213 | 221 | 228 | 235 | 242 | 250 | 258 | 265 |
| 204 | 212 | 219 | 227 | 235 | 242 | 250 | 257 | 265 | 272 |
| 210 | 218 | 225 | 233 | 241 | 249 | 256 | 264 | 272 | 280 |
| 216 | 224 | 232 | 240 | 248 | 256 | 264 | 272 | 279 | 287 |
| 221 | 230 | 238 | 246 | 254 | 263 | 271 | 279 | 287 | 295 |

## What's My Body Mass Index? continued

Locate your height in the left-hand column. Then move across until you find your weight. The number at the top of the column is your BMI. Pounds have been rounded off.

| BMI | 37 | 38 | 39 | 40 | 41 | 42 | 43 | 44 |
|---|---|---|---|---|---|---|---|---|
| Height (inches) | | | | Body Weight (pounds) | | | | |
| 58 | 177 | 181 | 186 | 191 | 196 | 201 | 205 | 210 |
| 59 | 183 | 188 | 193 | 198 | 203 | 208 | 212 | 217 |
| 60 | 189 | 194 | 199 | 204 | 209 | 215 | 220 | 225 |
| 61 | 195 | 201 | 206 | 211 | 217 | 222 | 227 | 232 |
| 62 | 202 | 207 | 213 | 218 | 224 | 229 | 235 | 240 |
| 63 | 208 | 214 | 220 | 225 | 231 | 237 | 242 | 248 |
| 64 | 215 | 221 | 227 | 232 | 238 | 244 | 250 | 256 |
| 65 | 222 | 228 | 234 | 240 | 246 | 252 | 258 | 264 |
| 66 | 229 | 235 | 241 | 247 | 253 | 260 | 266 | 272 |
| 67 | 236 | 242 | 249 | 255 | 261 | 268 | 274 | 280 |
| 68 | 243 | 249 | 256 | 262 | 269 | 276 | 282 | 289 |
| 69 | 250 | 257 | 263 | 270 | 277 | 284 | 291 | 297 |
| 70 | 257 | 264 | 271 | 278 | 285 | 292 | 299 | 306 |
| 71 | 265 | 272 | 279 | 286 | 293 | 301 | 308 | 315 |
| 72 | 272 | 279 | 287 | 294 | 302 | 309 | 316 | 324 |
| 73 | 280 | 288 | 295 | 302 | 310 | 318 | 325 | 333 |
| 74 | 287 | 295 | 303 | 311 | 319 | 326 | 334 | 342 |
| 75 | 295 | 303 | 311 | 319 | 327 | 335 | 343 | 351 |
| 76 | 304 | 312 | 320 | 328 | 336 | 344 | 353 | 361 |

| 45 | 46 | 47 | 48 | 49 | 50 | 51 | 52 | 53 | 54 |
|---|---|---|---|---|---|---|---|---|---|
| | | | | **Body Weight (pounds)** | | | | | |
| 215 | 220 | 224 | 229 | 234 | 239 | 244 | 248 | 253 | 258 |
| 222 | 227 | 232 | 237 | 242 | 247 | 252 | 257 | 262 | 267 |
| 230 | 235 | 240 | 245 | 250 | 255 | 261 | 266 | 271 | 276 |
| 238 | 243 | 248 | 254 | 259 | 264 | 269 | 275 | 280 | 285 |
| 246 | 251 | 256 | 262 | 267 | 273 | 278 | 284 | 289 | 295 |
| 254 | 259 | 265 | 270 | 278 | 282 | 287 | 293 | 299 | 304 |
| 262 | 267 | 273 | 279 | 285 | 291 | 296 | 302 | 308 | 314 |
| 270 | 276 | 282 | 288 | 294 | 300 | 306 | 312 | 318 | 324 |
| 278 | 284 | 291 | 297 | 303 | 309 | 315 | 322 | 328 | 334 |
| 287 | 293 | 299 | 306 | 312 | 319 | 325 | 331 | 338 | 344 |
| 295 | 302 | 308 | 315 | 322 | 328 | 335 | 341 | 348 | 354 |
| 304 | 311 | 318 | 324 | 331 | 338 | 345 | 351 | 358 | 365 |
| 313 | 320 | 327 | 334 | 341 | 348 | 355 | 362 | 369 | 376 |
| 322 | 329 | 338 | 343 | 351 | 358 | 365 | 372 | 379 | 386 |
| 331 | 338 | 346 | 353 | 361 | 368 | 375 | 383 | 390 | 397 |
| 340 | 348 | 355 | 363 | 371 | 378 | 386 | 393 | 401 | 408 |
| 350 | 358 | 365 | 373 | 381 | 389 | 396 | 404 | 412 | 420 |
| 359 | 367 | 375 | 383 | 391 | 399 | 407 | 415 | 423 | 431 |
| 369 | 377 | 385 | 394 | 402 | 410 | 418 | 426 | 435 | 443 |

Or, you can find the intersection of your height and weight in the chart on pages 8–11. You can also type "BMI calculator" into any search engine and find dozens of Web sites that will do the calculation for you.

If you're an NBA power forward or champion sprinter, you may discover — to your shock and horror — that your BMI falls above the healthy range. Do not head straight to your nearest Weight Watchers program! BMI measurements for very muscular people can be highly unreliable. That's because BMI, unlike body-fat tests (described in Question #8), doesn't distinguish between fat and muscle. For the average person, BMI does happen to correlate fairly well with body composition (the ratio of muscle to fat), but it doesn't work that way for muscular people. Under the current BMI guidelines, Arnold Schwarzenegger — at 6-foot-2 and 257 rock-solid pounds, with a BMI of 33 — is considered obese.

BMI is also unreliable for pregnant women because they're supposed to be carrying extra weight, and it may underestimate body fat in older people and others who have lost muscle mass.

Even if you're not pregnant or a professional athlete, don't place too much emphasis on your BMI. If you're a couch potato whose BMI falls into the healthy range, your score shouldn't give you license to maintain a slothful lifestyle. And if you're a regular exerciser with a high BMI, don't assume you're headed for trouble. There are plenty of "overweight" people who are healthy and metabolically normal. It's important to consider all of the health and fitness measures described in Question #1.

## Question #3: Are Americans really that much fatter than they used to be?

*The short answer:* Yep.

*Every ten years or so,* the federal government sends health professionals all over the country in mobile examination centers to measure, weigh, and extensively interview a sample of several thousand people who represent the American population. The results of this undertaking, called the National Health and Nutrition Examination Survey, show that our nation's waistbands are expanding significantly.

While the average height of Americans has remained the same for the past 50 years, our weight has increased. The government survey conducted from 1976 to 1980 found the average man to be 5-foot-9 and 172.2 pounds, and the average woman to be 5-foot-3½ and 144.4 pounds. In the next survey, taken from 1988 to 1994, the average man — no taller than in the previous survey — weighed in at 180 pounds, the average woman, still 5-foot-3½, weighed in at 152 pounds.

No height/weight data have been published since, but the government has issued body mass index numbers that show the steady fattening of America. From the first survey, completed in 1980, to the most recent, completed in 2000, the population considered overweight (BMI 25 or higher) or obese (BMI 30 or higher) increased from 47 percent to 64 percent. Over the same period, the obese category alone more than doubled, from 15 percent to 31 percent.

Is it because we're eating more or moving less? Probably both. In 2000, women ate on average 335 more calories per day than they did in 1971, according to the Centers for Disease Control. Men consumed 168 more daily calories than they did three decades earlier. CDC research shows that men now consume about 2,618 calories per day and women 1,877 calories. There's no precise data measuring changes in activity levels, but as we explain in Question #4, we're a lot less active than we used to be.

## Question #4: How much less active are we compared to our premodern ancestors?

*The short answer:* Those of us who live in the world of remote controls, video games, automobiles, elevators, dishwashers, and other modern conveniences probably burn 500 to 1,000 fewer calories per day than our ancestors who lived a few hundred years ago, according to studies of the Amish and some Australian actors.

*Unless someone invents a time-travel machine,* we'll never know for sure how much more active our ancestors were. But researchers in Australia made a creative attempt at calculating an estimate: They paid actors to live in huts for up to four days at "Old Sydney Days," a theme park set around the early nineteenth century. The actors — theme park employees who played the roles of early Australian soldiers, convicts, and settlers — wore devices that tracked their every move. The researchers compared the actors' activity levels with those of sedentary office workers.

As a group, the results showed, the seven actors walked approximately 5 miles a day more than their desk-jockey counterparts. But the two actors who took their roles most seriously, according to the researchers, walked about 10 miles a day more than the office workers.

This was a small study conducted under artificial conditions — the participants were hardly following the exact daily routines of nineteenth-century Australian settlers. But the results jibe with a study of a community that genuinely maintains old-fashioned ways: the Amish. University of Tennessee researchers equipped 98 Canadian Amish men and women with pedometers and recorded their activities in detail for one week as the Amish went about chopping wood, plowing their fields without modern machinery, and so on.

Among the findings: Amish men averaged 18,425 steps a day (about 9 miles) and reported 12 hours of walking a week. Amish women averaged 14,196 steps (about 7 miles) and reported 5.7 hours of walking a week. The activities of Amish men included 10 hours of vigorous physical activity each week and 42.8 hours of moderate physical activity. Women performed 2.4 hours of vigorous physical activity a week and 39.2 hours of moderate physical activity.

The researchers didn't track a control group of non-Amish, so it's not clear exactly how the horse-and-buggy crowd compares. But based on other research, the Amish are probably taking about 10,000 more steps per day than the rest of us, says study coauthor David Bassett, Ph.D., an exercise science professor at the University of Tennessee. "That would equate to about 5 more miles of walking," says Bassett, but "that's going to underestimate calories burned because a lot of their physical activity is upper body, which the pedometer won't pick up." Bassett estimates that the Amish are about six times more active than the average American and burn about 1,000 more calories per day.

Not surprisingly, they're a lot leaner, too. None of the Amish men met the criterion for obesity (BMI of 30), compared to 27.7 percent of American men as a whole. Among the women, 9 percent were obese, compared with 34 percent of American women.

## Question #5: Are Americans the fattest people in the world?

*The short answer:* Samoa wins the "globesity" contest, but the United States is the fattest industrialized nation on earth.

*Among the inhabitants of Samoa,* a cluster of islands in the South Pacific, more than 56 percent of the men and 74 percent of the women have a BMI over 30, the clinical definition of obesity.

Although Americans are still far behind Samoa, more than 30 percent are classified as obese and roughly another one-third are considered overweight. "Our obesity rates are nearly twice as high as [those in] Canada, Australia, and New Zealand," says Barry Popkin, Ph.D., director of nutritional epidemiology at the University of North Carolina at Chapel Hill. "They're almost three times higher than [those in] France, Spain, and the Netherlands."

Popkin warns that waistlines are expanding worldwide at an alarming rate. The nations that come closest to rivaling the United States, with average obesity rates in the teens, are Greece, Kuwait, Egypt, Germany, Mexico, and Finland. Even nations still considered slim and trim, such as Japan, China, and Peru, are beginning to put on weight. So many nations besides the United States have seen their obesity rates double in the last decade.

The reason for this global corpulence? According to Popkin:

## Samoa Wins the "Globesity" Contest

Here's a glance at some of the obesity rates around the world. Experts warn that waistlines are expanding at an alarming rate.

| Country | BMI 25–29.9 Male | BMI >30 Male | BMI 25–29.9 Female | BMI >30 Female |
| --- | --- | --- | --- | --- |
| Belgium | 49.0 | 14.0 | 28.0 | 13.0 |
| Canada | 41.5 | 11.0 | 35.6 | 13.0 |
| Chile | N/A | 15.7 | N/A | 23.0 |
| China | 2.3 | 1.0 | 14.4 | 1.7 |
| England | 46.6 | 21.0 | 32.0 | 23.0 |
| France | 29.0 | 12.0 | 29.0 | 17.0 |
| Germany | N/A | 18.0 | N/A | 20.0 |
| Greece | 45.0 | 29.0 | 41.0 | 28.0 |
| Italy | 41.0 | 9.5 | 26.0 | 9.9 |
| Japan | 24.3 | 1.9 | 20.2 | 3.4 |
| Samoa | N/A | 56.0 | N/A | 74.3 |
| Spain | 56.0 | 10.0 | 43.0 | 14.0 |
| Sweden | 41.0 | 10.0 | 30.0 | 12.0 |
| Switzerland | 33.0 | 6.0 | 17.0 | 5.0 |
| United States | 39.3 | 27.7 | 28.0 | 34.0 |

super-sizing, cheap and plentiful junk food, escalators, elevators, e-mail, remote controls, computer games — every advancement designed to make us eat more and/or move less. Many poorer nations have the added challenge of shifting abruptly from an agricultural to an industrial economy; practically overnight, entire populations go from tending the fields and eating taro root and fish to working desk jobs and eating Big Macs. Samoans and members of other societies may also be victims of their so-called "thrifty" genes, which historically helped them preserve body fat when food was scarce but work against them now that they subsist on a high-fat, high-calorie diet.

## Question #6: To what extent is my weight influenced by my genes?

*The short answer:* On average, research suggests, a person's weight is probably a bit more than 50 percent influenced by genetic factors. However, in certain populations the environment plays a larger role.

*When you see a family* in which every member is as slim as Lara Flynn Boyle, you may wonder: Are they svelte because they're genetically programmed to be or because they go on family hikes and never set foot in a Burger King? The influence of genetics and the environment on weight is an issue that scientists have been trying to sort out for decades.

A wealth of knowledge has come from research on identical twins, who, of course, share all the same genes. In a classic Canadian study published in the *New England Journal of Medicine,* researchers sequestered 12 sets of identical male twins for 100 days at a college dorm. Six days a week, the twins were fed 1,000 calories per day more than they needed to maintain their weight; other than walking for 30 minutes daily, the subjects performed virtually no physical activity. At the end of the study, each subject had consumed 84,000 extra calories — enough, theoretically, to gain about 24 pounds (since it generally takes an extra 3,500 calories to gain 1 pound of fat). But that's not what happened: Some men gained as little as 9.5 pounds, whereas others gained as much as 29 pounds. The difference in weight gain *among* the various twin pairs was three times greater than the average difference *within* the pairs. The location of the extra fat deposited — whether below the waist, deep in the belly, or beneath the skin in the abdominal area — also was similar within the pairs but varied greatly between pairs.

Research comparing twins raised apart and twins raised together confirms the significant influence of genes on body fat. In a study of some 600 Swedish twins, the body mass index scores of identical twins raised apart were just as similar as BMI scores of identical twins raised together. And the BMI scores within the identical twin pairs were far more similar than the BMI scores within the fraternal twin pairs. The researchers concluded that, at least in Western society, genetic factors may account for as much as 70 percent of weight differences among individuals.

So does this mean your weight is essentially predetermined? Absolutely not. Sure, if you're genetically susceptible to obesity and your idea of a workout is lifting the lid off a bucket of KFC chicken, you will likely be heavier than a fellow couch potato/KFC fiend who has a propensity to be lean. But if you take up cycling and switch from fried chicken drumsticks to skinless baked breasts, you're likely to stay at a healthy weight regardless of your genes. "Someone who has a susceptibility toward obesity just has to be more careful," says Tracy Nelson, Ph.D., MPH, a University of Colorado expert on gene-environment interactions in the development of obesity.

Clearly, the rising obesity levels over the last generation (see Question #3) show that eating habits and activity levels can drastically affect body weight. Our genes haven't changed that fast, but our environment has.

In certain regions, environmental influences are expressed more fully than in others. For instance, it is primarily lifestyle differences that explain why only 13.8 percent of Colorado residents are obese, compared with 24.3 percent of Mississippians. However, it is largely genetic differences that explain why certain Native American populations have higher obesity rates than other Americans with similar habits.

## Question #7: Am I destined to gain fat and lose muscle mass as I get older?

*The short answer:* Not necessarily. If you start when you're young, you can prevent most of the muscle atrophy and fat gain commonly associated with aging by committing to both weight training and aerobic exercise. Although it's difficult to reverse a near-lifetime of sedentary habits, even older exercisers can make significant health and fitness improvements with a fitness program begun in middle age.

*With age many changes are inevitable:* Your hair will turn gray, your skin will wrinkle, and you'll berate your grandchildren for not calling often enough. You'll probably start thinking Regis Philbin is handsome, too. But saddlebags and a spare tire are *not* a given. Neither, for the most part, is muscle shrinkage. Although some muscle loss and fat gain (especially in postmenopausal women) may be unavoidable, most of the physical decline and waistline expansion considered to be a normal part of aging is actually due to chronic inactivity, a.k.a. sitting on your butt watching the Food Network.

Cardiovascular exercise is important for weight control because it's the type of exercise that burns the most calories. However, walking on the treadmill isn't enough. The key to maintaining your svelteness and your strength as you get older is lifting weights. That's right: Even if you enjoy jogging or swimming, you need to make the acquaintance of some dumbbells. Without weight training, most people lose 30 percent to 40 percent of their muscle between the ages of 30 and 70; as a result, they experience a metabolic slowdown and pack on pounds more easily. In one study, very experienced swimmers and runners around age 70 were found to have about the same amount of muscle mass as sedentary people their age. However, 70-year-olds who had lifted weights regularly for more than a decade were as packed with muscle as 28-year-olds.

The bottom line: If you want to spend your golden years looking like Jack LaLanne instead of Marlon Brando, get thee to a weight room. And to a treadmill, too.

## Question #8: Should I get my body fat tested?

*The short answer:* If you're trying to slim down, a body-fat test is a better gauge of your progress than a scale and it can help you set realistic weight goals. However, as we explain in Question #1, your total body fat doesn't tell you that much about your health or fitness.

*A body-fat test,* also known as a body-composition test, tells you how much of your weight is composed of fat and how much is composed of lean body mass — muscle, bones, blood, water, organs, and connective tissue. There are more than a half dozen testing methods, ranging in cost from $25 to $100.

What's a good score? Experts disagree on the precise numbers, but the general consensus is that men should not exceed 20 percent to 22 percent body fat. For women, the high end of healthy is somewhere between 26 percent and 30 percent, although some experts believe that women who exercise and eat healthfully are not at increased risk for disease until they hit 35 percent fat. Women begin to see muscle definition once they dip below about 22 percent body fat, and men start to look more ripped when they drop to less than about 15 percent body fat.

Because your disease risk is influenced by the location of your fat (see Question #13) and other factors, it's impossible to equate a body-fat score with increased risk of disease. A woman who is 30 percent fat but walks daily and carries the bulk of her fat in her hips or thighs is likely to be at lower risk for diabetes and heart disease than a sedentary woman who is 30 percent fat and carries more fat in her abdominal area. (Also, "fat" women who are active and fit are generally healthier and have lower death rates than leaner women who are sedentary and unfit.)

Maybe you can never be too rich, but you can definitely be too thin, and a body-fat test can also reveal whether you are in this unhealthy category. Women who don't have enough body fat stop menstruating, a serious condition called *amenorrhea* that can lead to thinning bones and other health problems. In general, women who are below 20 percent fat are at greater risk for amenorrhea, although some women don't stop menstruating until they hit 16 or even 14 percent fat. Men also need a certain amount of body fat for the protection of vital organs, proper body temperature regulation, and countless other functions. Experts put the low end of the healthy range for men at 8 percent, although many elite male athletes have even less.

Body-fat tests show how meaningless a person's scale weight can be. Two women who are 5-foot-7 and weigh 150 pounds might look very different, depending on their body composition. One may be a tennis player with rock-hard muscles and 18 percent body fat; the other may be an eBay addict who bids on exercise equipment but never actually purchases any — and as a result is a soft, squishy 30 percent body fat.

Knowing your body composition can give you a rational basis for choosing a weight goal, as opposed to picking a weight out of thin air, as many people do. For instance, if you're a woman and a body-fat test reveals that you have 115 pounds of lean body mass, it will be obvious that your weight goal of 125 pounds is highly unrealistic, not to mention unhealthy. Although you inevitably lose some muscle as you drop fat, the weight of your bones, organs, and other lean body tissue isn't going to change. With roughly 115 pounds of lean tissue, your dream weight of 125 would put you somewhere around 8 percent body fat — far, far too low for a woman.

If you're trying to lose weight, getting your body fat tested every six months is a good way to monitor your progress. (Don't get tested more frequently because, unlike scales, body-fat tests aren't sensitive to small changes.) A body-composition test is more useful than the scale because it distinguishes fat loss from muscle or water loss. If you're on a weight-loss plan that doesn't include strength training, a good portion of the weight you lose is likely to be muscle, so your scale weight may overstate your progress.

On the other hand, if lifting weights is part of your program, you may be discouraged by the numbers on the scale. Despite all your efforts to trim calories and work out, your weight may barely decrease — or may even stay the same or nudge upward. This, of course, is because muscle is denser than fat. A body-fat test may help gauge your true progress. Whereas the scale might say you've lost 1 pound, a body-fat test might tell you that you've actually lost 4 pounds of fat while gaining 3 pounds of fat-free mass. A body-fat test can be proof of your progress when the scale suggests otherwise.

Still, as we explain in Questions 9 and 10, no body-fat testing method is entirely accurate, so don't take your results too literally. If, after embarking on an exercise program, you feel better and your clothes fit better, that may be a more useful gauge of your progress than the results of a body-fat test.

## Question #9: What's the most accurate way to get my body fat tested?

*The short answer:* There are three methods considered to be the most accurate: underwater weighing, an x-ray body scan called DEXA, and an egg-shaped chamber called the BOD POD. However, these methods are less accessible to the general public than the less reliable methods described in Question #10.

*Although underwater weighing* has long been considered the gold standard in body-fat testing, with a margin of error of 2 to 3 percentage points, a pile of research has found DEXA and the BOD POD to be equally accurate. This is good news, since underwater weighing is about as much fun as having a colonoscopy. Here's a rundown of the three most accurate methods.

### Underwater Weighing

You step into a tank of water, blow out as much air as possible, then sit on an underwater scale. While submerged, you expel even more air, until you feel like your lungs are about to explode. Your weight underwater is used to calculate your body composition and body density. Fat is less dense than water, whereas muscle is denser; the more fat you have, the more your body wants to float when dunked under water. This method will overestimate your fat if you fail to blow out all your air and may slightly underestimate the fat content of people who have dense bones. You can get tested at some university labs (call the exercise physiology department), and a company called FitnessWave (getdunked.com) has a tank inside of a truck that travels to health clubs in the western United States.

## DEXA (Dual X-Ray Absorptiometry)

With this test, offered by some hospitals, you lie on a platform for 5 to 20 minutes while very low doses of two different x-ray energies scan your body. Originally developed to measure bone density, DEXA determines not just your body-fat percentage but also the location of your fat. This is helpful because abdominal fat poses a greater health risk than fat in the hips and thighs (Question #13 explains why). DEXA is especially useful for people with below- or above-average bone density because it's the only method that calculates bone mass and soft-tissue mass separately. The other methods lump both types of lean mass together, so a person with denser bones may appear leaner than he or she actually is, and vice versa.

## The BOD POD

Wearing a swimsuit and a swim cap and feeling fairly silly, you step on a scale and then sit in a sealed 5-foot-tall, white, egg-shaped chamber that looks like something out of *Star Trek: The Next Generation*. Computerized pressure sensors determine how much fat and muscle you have by measuring the amount of air your body displaces. (This is similar to the concept of underwater weighing, which measures how much water your body displaces, but the process is much quicker and you don't have to get your hair wet.) It's crucial to cover your hair with a swim cap and to wear nothing but a swimsuit because hair and clothing can trap air, causing the machine to underestimate your body fat. Body hair and facial hair in men have been shown to skew the results by ½ to 1 percent beyond the normal 2 to 3 percent margin of error. The BOD POD (bodpod.com) is available primarily at universities and hospitals, although some gyms have made the investment.

## Question #10: What's the most convenient way to get my body fat tested?

*The short answer:* Two methods you're most likely to come across are skinfold calipers and bioelectrical impedance (the technology behind body-fat scales). Although these methods aren't inherently the most accurate, you can take precautions to make the results more trustworthy.

### Skinfold Calipers

Skinfold calipers, commonly used by fitness trainers and registered dietitians, look something like spring-loaded lobster claws. The tester pinches three to seven spots on your body, and a gauge measures each hunk of flesh in millimeters. The tester then plugs the results into an equation.

Calipers can be accurate within 4 percentage points, but only if the tester is skilled at separating fat from muscle and pinches precisely the right spots. Even experienced testers can have difficulty testing subjects who have taut skin, especially on the thighs; considerable excess fat, especially in the abdominal area; or highly developed muscles. Also, accuracy may depend on the equation used, as different racial groups tend to carry fat in different places. And it's important that the tester use a formula that takes age into consideration. Fat tends to move inward with age, but calipers pinch only fat near the skin; so, unless the tester uses a formula designed for seniors, the amount of fat pinched by the caliper in an older person might underestimate the person's total body fat.

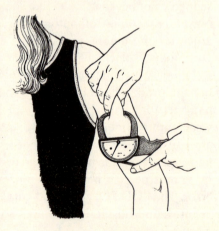

*Large skinfold calipers*

You can purchase do-it-yourself calipers over the Internet for less than $20, but you won't get as accurate a reading as a trained professional would, and some experts think they're too inaccurate to be of any use.

## Bioelectrical Impedance

Bioelectrical impedance is a quick, painless method that comes in three varieties: full body, lower body (such as the Tanita scale), and upper body (hand-held devices such as the Omron Body Logic). With full-body impedance, offered by some trainers and nutritionists, you lie on your back while an electrical signal travels from an electrode on your foot to an electrode on your hand. The faster the signal, the more muscular you are. This is because water conducts electricity, and muscle is 70 percent water; fat contains a lot less water, so it "impedes" the signal.

When you step on a body-fat scale, a signal travels through your lower body, from one foot to the other. When you hold the Omron, a plastic gizmo that looks like half of a car steering wheel, the signal shoots through your upper body, from hand to hand. Even under optimal conditions, the margin of error for full-body impedance is about 4 percent and perhaps 1 percentage point more for the scale or upper-body devices. Since many people don't experience changes in body fat of this magnitude, impedance methods may have a margin of error that's too high to accurately detect body-fat changes for the average person. What's more, impedance gadgets are highly sensitive to hydration status. If you're dehydrated, the test can overestimate your body fat by as much as 10 percentage points. Also, impedance devices are typically less accurate for people who are obese or very lean. For best results, get tested first thing in the morning, before you've eaten or exercised but after you've normalized your hydration status with a glass of water. Women should avoid testing during menstruation because some retain water during that time.

## Question #11: If I gain weight, will I gain fat cells or will the ones I have expand?

*The short answer:* For the most part, you stretch out your existing fat cells when you gain weight, although under certain circumstances you may also gain new fat cells.

*Your fat cells,* known as adipocytes, multiply in number when you're a baby and during puberty. You can also produce new fat cells during pregnancy or if you weigh at least 200 percent more than a healthy body weight. There is also some evidence that even people of normal weight may gain some fat cells as they age. In general, however, weight gain is primarily due to existing fat cells plumping up.

When you lose weight, your fat cells shrink, but you're stuck with the same number. Most people have between 25 and 35 billion fat cells, and women have more than men. Some obese people have as many as 75 billion. Scientists think that the more adipocytes you have, the more difficult it is to lose weight and the harder it is to maintain weight loss.

The only way to decrease your fat cell count is to have liposuction. Once you've had fat cells sucked out of you, they don't grow back, although your remaining cells can certainly fatten up.

## Question #12: What exactly is cellulite?

*The short answer:* It's garden-variety body fat that's stored a bit differently than fat in other places on your body.

*Cottage cheese.* Orange-peel skin. Golf-ball butt. Derrière dimples. These are just some of the nicknames we have for the much-maligned bumpiness beneath the surface of the skin, primarily in the hip and thigh area. Although weight-loss product manufacturers would have you believe cellulite is a unique kind of fat that's responsive to special treatments, in reality it's your basic body fat. The reason it has a ripply appearance is that it's compartmentalized by connective tissue called collagen. To get a super-magnified idea of why cellulite is bumpy, press your arm against a chainlink fence and watch how your skin bulges through the openings.

About 85 percent of women and a small fraction of men develop cellulite after puberty. Even some lean and muscular women have it. There are several theories about what causes cellulite to form, but most experts think it's a combination of hormones, genetics, and excess body fat. There's no reliable, nonsurgical method to rid yourself of the ripples, although the leaner you are, the less likely you are to have dimples on your derrière.

## Question #13: Is it true that a beer belly is more unhealthy than saddlebags?

*The short answer:* Yes. Much above-the-waist fat is stored deep within the gut, clustered around vital organs, where it can wreak havoc on blood-cholesterol levels and cause other problems. Hip and thigh fat, on the other hand, sits just underneath the skin and more or less stays out of circulation. Not only that, it may actually take some of your blood fats out of circulation.

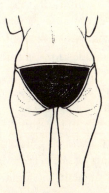

*A beer belly is more unhealthy than saddlebags.*

*When you have excess fat cells* deep in the abdominal region — fat cells that are highly active — you have more fat molecules traveling to the liver, where they're repackaged and sent out to clog the arteries in the form of triglycerides and LDL cholesterol (the "bad" cholesterol). Thigh fat cells, on the other hand, operate at a less frenetic pace; when fat molecules arrive in the thighs, they settle in for a good while. This isn't great news if you want slimmer hips — thigh fat is very stubborn — but it does mean you have less fat circulating in the bloodstream. And if it's any consolation, sporting a little extra in the legs and butt may offer protection from heart disease.

Research shows that for both men and women, fat seems to migrate inward with age. This can be problematic, since ab fat has also been linked to insulin resistance (defined in Question #211) and high blood pressure (explained in Question #28). Exercise appears to prevent some, but probably not all, of the age-related increase in fat that lies deep within the gut.

## Question #14: Does muscle really weigh more than fat?

*The short answer:* Sort of.

*Actually, this is the wrong way to phrase the question.* It's like asking if a pound of gold weighs more than a pound of feathers. Of course, the answer is that a pound is a pound is a pound, no matter what substance you place on the scale. Here's a better way to ask this question: Is muscle denser than fat? To that question, the answer is yes.

Density refers to how much space something takes up. The denser an object, the less room it consumes per pound. Obviously, a pound of gold takes up less space than a pound of feathers. Well, think of muscle as gold and fat as feathers: A pound of muscle takes up about 22 percent less space than a pound of fat. This explains why a lean, muscular bodybuilder performing great feats of strength on ESPN may weigh the same as the pudgy, Fritos-scarfing couch potato who watches him on the boob tube.

This also explains why stepping on a scale is a poor way to determine whether you are too fat or whether your weight-loss program is working. A traditional scale does not distinguish between fat weight and muscle weight. If your new fitness program includes weight training (as it should), you may find that your scale weight creeps up by a pound or two but your clothes are looser. This likely means that you've added dense, space-efficient muscle to your frame while you've lost space-hogging fat.

### Question #15: If I stop exercising, will my muscles turn to fat?

*The short answer:* No.

*This myth has prevailed* in part because many former athletes who were once buff and brawny begin to resemble Santa Claus as they get older. This doesn't mean that their muscle has "turned into fat" any more than it means that their muscle has turned into wood, stone, or chocolate pudding. Muscle is muscle and fat is fat. You can't magically transform one type of tissue into another.

The aging former athletes who plump up do so for the same reason everyone else gets fat: They stop exercising and start eating too much. Their muscles gradually shrink from neglect while their body-fat stores expand from consuming excess calories.

If for some reason you stop exercising, the muscle you've built up will slowly atrophy. If you cut back on calories accordingly, you probably won't gain fat, but you certainly won't look as tight and firm as you did in more active times. If you happen to have a lifestyle that's completely sedentary and frequently utter the words "Extra mayo, please," you're likely to gain significant amounts of fat as well.

Question #16: I seem to weigh more when my scale is on a carpet than when it's on tile. Am I imagining this?

*The short answer:* Nope. A scale's fulcrums — internal gizmos that resemble mini–suspension bridges — don't bend as much on carpets as they do on hard surfaces, so your weight may appear to be slightly higher on your shag rug.

*Physicists from a British university* positioned six standard analog scales on different surfaces and discovered a whopping 10 percent increase in weight when the scale was placed on a thick carpet, compared with a wood or tile floor. That's because on a hard surface, the base of the scale bows inward, which shortens the distance between the scale's fulcrums, the tiny levers placed at each corner to transmit weight to the spring-loaded metal plate on the back of the scale.

Place the scale on deep carpet, and the scale sinks into it. Because the base is supported, it doesn't bend, thereby increasing the distance between the fulcrums. Even a small increase can add several pounds to the weight registered on the display. Most manufacturers calibrate their scales on hard surfaces.

The British researchers also found that digital scales, which use a different internal mechanism, were far less prone to variances when placed on different surfaces. However, when the floor was not completely level, the displayed weights of all types of scales varied, fluctuating up or down depending on how the floor sloped.

Question #17: I've heard there are three distinct body types. What are they, and why do they matter?

*The short answer:* Although there are countless variations on each, most bodies fall into some variation of three broad categories: ectomorphs, endomorphs, and mesomorphs. Knowing this can give you some insight on the type of results you can expect to see from your training program.

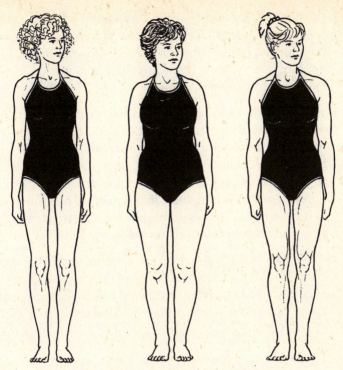

*Most people fall into one of three general body types:
ectomorph, endomorph, or mesomorph.*

*Your body's structural blueprint* is determined even before you are born. Although exercise and diet can change your body-fat percentage and, to some extent, the size of your muscles, your basic structure will always remain the same (unless, of course, you have Michael Jackson's addiction to plastic surgery). This is a tough fact for some people to accept. But if you've spent a lifetime — and a fortune — trying to achieve a body for which you are simply not designed, we think it should be considered a welcome relief from the frustration. Here's a look at the characteristics of the three main body types.

*Ectomorphs* are long, wiry, and narrow. They generally have delicate bone structures, and their shoulders and hips are approximately the same width. Accomplished long-distance runners, ballerinas, and basketball players are often ecto-morphs. Famous ectomorphs include Michelle Pfeiffer, Whit-ney Houston, Manute Bol, Chris Rock, and just about every model to strut down the runway.

*Endomorphs* are soft, curvy, and often pear-shaped: that is, their hips are wider than their shoulders. Though this body type holds on to fat a little more tenaciously than the other two, many famous actresses and singers are wonderful ex-amples of how sexy and curvaceous endos can be. Jennifer Lopez, Oprah Winfrey, and Cindy Crawford are examples of fit endomorphs. Male endomorphs are somewhat rare, since men tend to carry less body fat below the belt than women.

*Mesomorphs* have big bones and tend to muscle-up easily. Their shoulders are often wider than their hips, and they are often described as having "medium" builds. Think sprinters, soccer players, and tennis players. Madonna, Tina Turner, Russell Crowe, and Vin Diesel are all fit mesomorphs.

## Question #18: Where does the word *muscle* come from?

*The short answer: Muscle* comes from the Latin word *mus,* which means "mouse." The way the muscles moved under the skin re-minded early scientists of a mouse moving.

## Question #19: I hear athletes and sports commentators talk about fast-twitch and slow-twitch muscle fibers. What do these terms mean?

*The short answer:* They're the two types of muscle fibers in the human body. Your ratio of fast-twitch to slow-twitch fibers in large part determines whether you're more suited for running the 100-meter dash or swimming the English Channel.

*If your lifelong fantasy* is sprinting to a world record in that 100-meter dash, you'd better have been born with plenty of fast-twitch muscle fibers. These fibers fire with lightening speed — about 50 milliseconds per contraction, compared with the 110 milliseconds it takes for slow-twitch muscle fibers to contract. They're good at tapping into your body's stored energy and don't need oxygen to operate. They're the first muscles called upon when you spring into action, and they're the ones that provide the brawn for short, explosive bursts of movement like sprinting, jumping, and swinging a golf club. They're also the first muscle fibers to poop out, which is why you don't see many world-class sprinters switching to ultra-marathons.

Slow-twitch muscle fibers are more like the Energizer Bunny: Once they fire up, they keep going and going and going. Slow-twitch fibers, which need oxygen to function, are the fibers you rely on to power long-distance runs and other slow, steady activities such as strolling through the park, ironing, and standing in line for the latest blockbuster movie.

With the right training program, you can improve your performance in just about any type of athletic event, but your potential is limited by, among other things, the percentage of each fiber type you're born with. Champion sprinters have about a 80:20 ratio of fast-twitch to slow-twitch fibers; elite distance runners have roughly an 80:20 slow-to-fast ratio. The average person has roughly a 50:50 ratio. Scientists have found that you can coax a certain percentage of your fast-twitch fibers to behave more like slow-twitch fibers by doing regular long-lasting, low-intensity workouts, but if you're built like a shot-putter, don't expect to be transformed into a Tour de France competitor.

How do you know what percentage of each type of muscle fibers you have? It's not information you really need, but if you have a burning desire to know, you can get a muscle biopsy. A lab technician will stick a large, thin needle into several of your muscles and then examine the extracted fibers under the microscope. A more pain-free, if less accurate, way to tell is to make an educated guess. If you have a predominance of fast-twitch muscles, you probably develop muscle easily and excel at sports that require fast reactions, good jumping ability, and keen hand-eye coordination. You've got a larger percentage of slow-twitch muscle if you have to work at building muscle but shine at endurance events.

## Question #20: What does the term *major muscle groups* mean?

*The short answer:* These are your larger muscles — and the ones that are the most important to target in your strength-training workouts. This term is used frequently in fitness magazines.

*Nobody expects you to do exercises* for each of the 650 muscles in your body, but it's a good idea to regularly work all of your major muscle groups: upper back, chest, shoulders, biceps, triceps, abdominals, lower back, buttocks, quadriceps, hamstrings, and calves. If you focus on these muscles, you'll likely hit most of your smaller, deeper muscles, which assist their larger colleagues in making movement happen.

## Question #21: In the gym I hear people throw around terms like *lats, delts, quads,* and *glutes*. What do these words mean?

*The short answer:* These are the slang terms for some of your major muscle groups. Veteran weightlifters like to toss these terms around, and you can, too, using the handy chart on page 37.

## Question #22: What is the strongest muscle in the body?

*The short answer:* It depends upon how you interpret the word *strong.*

*The masseter,* found on either side of your jaw, is the muscle that can generate the largest measurable force. Since it is very short and wide, it benefits from a mechanical advantage that many other muscles don't enjoy; in other words, it doesn't have to move very far to exert a force. This is the same reason someone with shorter arms may be able to lift a heavier weight than someone with similar muscle strength but longer limbs. Their arms don't have to move as far, so they don't have to exert as much effort.

According to the *Guinness Book of World Records,* one man with a highly developed set of masseter muscles achieved a bite strength of 975 pounds for two seconds. (Bite strength is measured with a device called a gnathodynamometer, which is sort of a plate with pressure sensors that you put in your mouth.) That's more than six times the typical biting strength of a human.

Most other muscles have a smaller point of attachment to the bone, which means they're more likely to tear under stress than the mighty masseter and also have much less leverage. If you could somehow detach your muscles from your bones and measure how much they could lift on their own, without the bones to help, the masseter would lose out against a lot of other muscles. The two top contenders, according to this interpretation, are the gluteus maximus — once again, size does matter — and the quadriceps (front thigh) muscles.

Some people claim the heart is "strongest" because it does more work over a lifetime than any other muscle, and it's almost impossible to fatigue. However, this isn't exactly a fair comparison, since the heart consists of a type of muscle that contracts whether you tell it to or not, whereas your masseter, glutes, and quadriceps are made up of a completely different variety of muscle, which contracts voluntarily.

## Question #23: What's the largest muscle in the body?

*The short answer:* Turn your head, look behind you, and glance down — you're staring right at it: the gluteus maximus, also known as your butt.

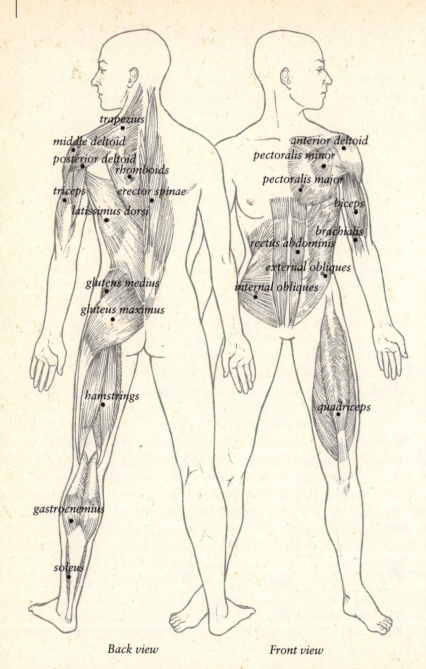

Back view

Front view

## Meet Your Muscles

Here's a brief rundown of your major muscle groups, including their formal names, nicknames, and job descriptions, along with a sampling of strength-training exercises that target them.

| Muscle Group | Formal Name | Nickname | Job Description | Classic Exercises |
|---|---|---|---|---|
| Upper back | Latissimus dorsi | Lats | Helping you pull | Lat pulldown, seated row, dumbbell row |
| Chest | Pectorals | Pecs | Helping you push | Bench press, vertical chest press, dumbbell fly |
| Shoulder | Deltoids | Delts | Helping move your arm in just about every direction | Overhead press, front raise, lateral raise |
| Upper arm, front | Biceps | Bis | Bending your arm at the elbow | Biceps curl, concentration curl, arm curl |
| Upper arm, rear | Triceps | Tris | Straightening your arm at the elbow | Triceps kickback, triceps press-down, French curl |
| Midsection | Abdominals (rectus abdominis, internal obliques, external obliques, transversus abdominis) | Abs | Bending your torso forward from the waist, twisting, stabilizing your body when you move other muscles | Ball crunch, bicycle, reverse crunch |
| Lower back | Erector spinae | None (sadly, these aren't popular muscles) | Helping with backward bending movements that involve tilting your pelvis forward; also, helping your abs stabilize your torso | Pelvic tilt, back raise |
| Buttocks | Gluteus maximus | Glutes | Helping you stand up from a seated position | Squat, lunge, leg press |
| Thigh, front | Quadriceps | Quads | Straightening your leg from the knee | Leg extension, squat, leg press |
| Thigh, rear | Hamstrings | Hams, hammies | Bending your knee and helping your glutes extend your hip | Leg curl, dead lift, lunge |
| Calf | Gastrocnemius and soleus | Calves | Raising you up on your tiptoes | Standing calf raise, seated calf raise |

*Your two "glutes" are responsible* for extending your hip. For example, when you get up out of a chair, it's your glutes, along with your thigh muscles, that help you stand up.

In case you were wondering, your longest muscle is your sartorius, a muscle that runs along the side of your leg from the middle of your hipbone to below your knee. Your sartorius is responsible for helping to flex and rotate both the hip and the knee.

## Question #24: What's the smallest muscle in the body?

*The short answer:* Your smallest muscles are your stapedius, which measures ½0 inch and activates your ear's "stirrup" in order to send vibrations from the eardrum to the inner ear, and the tiny muscles located in your eyes that help you focus. What these eye muscles lack in size, they make up for in ambition: They move about 100,000 times every day.

*The smallest muscles* that are worthy of some attention in the weight room reside in your fingers. These muscles, with such names as extensor digitorum communis and lumbricalis, are responsible for the subtle, precise movements your fingers are capable of, like playing the piano or untangling a necklace chain, as well as strength-oriented tasks such as gripping and holding. Even if you don't make a habit of climbing rocks or swinging on the parallel bars, strengthen-

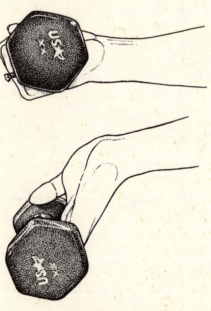

*Finger curls*

ing your finger muscles is a good idea. You'll develop more oomph for everything from twisting the cap off a beer to holding on to the bench press bar.

Strengthening your fingers doesn't require much time. You can buy some exercise putty to squish with your fingers as you talk on the phone or sit through your boss's weekly update meeting. You can also do finger curls: Hold a dumbbell in your hand, and sit in a chair with your legs apart. Lean forward and rest your right forearm on your right thigh so that your wrist hangs off the edge in front of your knee. Curl your wrist down and let the weight roll down into your fingertips. Hold a moment, then roll the weight up your fingers and curl your wrist upward. Then switch sides. Do one to three sets of 8 to 15 repetitions two or three times a week.

## Question #25: How many bones are there in the human body?

*The short answer:* As adults, we have 206 distinct bones in our bodies. However, newborn babies have about 350 bones, many of which fuse together by age 12.

## Question #26: Is it true that I'm taller in the morning than later in the day?

*The short answer:* Yes.

*Each vertebra in your spine* sits on a cushiony pad of cartilage known as a disk. While you sleep, these disks fill up with fluids and plump up like tiny water balloons. All of this extra fluid adds an extra bit of height to your stature, as much as half an inch. As the day goes on, these fluids seep out of your disks and into your bloodstream, the spaces of the vertebrae themselves, and other parts of the spinal column.

By the way, the extra fluid in your disks is one more reason to be very careful if you stretch right after you wake up. Until you move around, stimulating your spinal fluids to circulate again, your spine will be stiffer than it is later on. You should always warm up for a few minutes before you stretch, but that advice is doubly important to follow if you stretch first thing in the morning.

## Question #27: What exactly is blood pressure?

*The short answer:* It's a measure of how much pressure is placed on the walls of your heart as it beats and relaxes between beats.

*Do you know your blood pressure?* Most people don't, even though it's a critical measure of your risk for heart attack and stroke. And although "high blood pressure" is a term frequently tossed around in the media and doctors on *ER* are always saying things like, "BP: 150 over 90!" many people are unfamiliar with what exactly "blood pressure" means.

Blood pressure consists of two measurements: systolic and diastolic. Systolic measures how much pressure it takes to force blood out of your heart each time it contracts. Diastolic measures how much pressure there is in the walls of the heart as it relaxes between contractions. If your systolic is 122 and your diastolic is 70, your blood pressure is written as 122/70.

In case you're wondering, the gizmo that medical professionals use to take your blood pressure — the large mercury thermometer on wheels with a nylon cuff, a rubber bulb, and metal valve attached — is called a sphygmomanometer (pronounced SVIG-mo-MAN-nah-meter). The nurse or doctor wraps the cuff snugly around your upper arm, then places the flat end of a stethoscope against the artery located in the crook of your arm. With the ear buds placed in her ears so she can "listen" for your blood pressure, she then closes the valve and pumps air into the cuff by squeezing the bulb a few times. Once the cuff is fully pumped, she releases the valve slightly and listens for a series of small thumping beats. The first beat she hears is your systolic pressure; the last she hears is your diastolic.

To get the most accurate reading possible, don't exercise or ingest caffeine for at least four hours beforehand. Avoid getting yelled at by your boss, too, since stress can cause a spike in blood pressure. Some people get a high reading simply in response to seeing a nurse or physician, a reaction called "white coat syndrome." Many medications, even if they're bought over the counter, can also raise or lower your reading. If you get a high reading, this doesn't necessarily mean you have high blood pressure. It's best to get several readings over the course of a week or so to help identify your general blood-pressure range.

By the way, those automatic blood-pressure machines you can buy in drugstores don't give very precise readings, probably because they're sensitive to the slightest movement or difference in the placement of the cuff on your arm. Skip the machines you see in the mall that take your blood pressure for a quarter; they're also subject to wild inaccuracies.

## Question #28: How do I know if I have high blood pressure?

*The short answer:* High blood pressure, also known as hypertension, is defined as a consistent reading of greater than 140/90. Often called the "silent killer," it has no symptoms but is strongly associated with heart disease, stroke, and kidney failure.

*You have high blood pressure* if either your systolic or your diastolic is high — or, of course, if both are high. The only accurate way to know whether you have high blood pressure is to get it checked by a trained and experienced professional, usually a nurse or a physician, although some personal trainers have earned certifications that include in-depth blood-pressure training.

You're at increased risk for high blood pressure if you are over 35, obese, don't exercise much, are under constant high stress, and drink an excessive amount of alcohol or if high blood pressure runs in your family. African Americans and postmenopausal women also have a greater incidence of high blood pressure.

If you do have high blood pressure, your doctor will probably recommend that you make some changes in your lifestyle, such as losing weight, limiting the sodium and saturated fat in your diet, and starting an exercise program. (Heavy weightlifting may be off-limits, however, since it can cause temporary but large spikes in blood pressure.) You might also be put on blood-pressure-lowering medication and asked to have your blood pressure taken regularly. The more enlightened your physician is, the more likely he or she is to suggest meditation, relaxation, yoga, tai chi, or some other stress-reducing activity that has been shown to help reduce blood pressure.

Recently the National Heart, Lung, and Blood Institute created a new red-flag category for blood pressure called "high normal." This is defined as 130 to 139 for systolic blood pressure and 85 to 89 for diastolic blood pressure. If you fall into this category, you should consult with your physician about which blood-pressure-lowering strategies are best for you.

# Calorie Burning: Myths and Truths About Metabolism

What do Americans wish for most? Sure, we're all hoping for world peace, an end to global warming, and an economic boom. And winning the lottery wouldn't hurt, either. But if pollsters included "a faster metabolism" as an option in their surveys, it might rank right up there on the nationwide wish list. Given the number of diets, supplements, and exercise programs that promise to "fire up your metabolism!" and transform you into a "calorie-burning machine at any age!" it seems the public has a burning desire to burn more calories.

But what really works? What does metabolism even mean? And what exactly is a calorie, anyway? With a working knowledge of these terms, you'll be well equipped to distinguish the hype about calorie burning from the legitimate promises. In this section we put to rest some common misconceptions about the most and least effective ways to burn calories. Did you ever wonder which cardio machine burns the most calories? Or how much extra muscle it really takes to rev up your metabolism? You'll find the answers here.

The number of calories you burn in a day is, to a large extent, within your power. This section is full of advice and information that will help you maximize that number.

## Question #29: What exactly is a calorie?

*The short answer:* A calorie is a measure of energy. In technical terms, it's the amount of energy it takes to raise the temperature of 1 gram of water 1 degree Celsius (1.8 degrees Fahrenheit).

*Although we tend to associate* the term *calorie* with food and exercise, it's a measure that applies to anything containing energy. A gallon of gas, for instance, contains 31 million calories' worth of energy. When applied to food and exercise, energy is actually measured in kilocalories; there are 1,000 calories in 1 kilocalorie. So that pat of butter you count as 100 calories is, in reality, 100,000 calories. (Maybe if that number were posted on food labels, we'd think twice about eating so much!) Outside of scientific journals, kilocalories are usually referred to simply as calories, although sometimes on food labels a capital "C" is used instead of a small "c" to indicate a reference to kilocalories.

Those 100 calories' worth of energy you get from a pat of butter constitute roughly the same amount of energy it takes to power the average person on a 1-mile walk. When you burn off more calories than you eat, you lose weight; when you eat more than you burn, the excess calories are stored in the form of body fat.

## Question #30: How many calories do you have to burn to lose a pound of fat?

*The short answer:* To lose one pound of fat, you need to create a deficit of about 3,500 calories. In other words, you have to either burn 3,500 extra calories through exercise or cut 3,500 calories from your diet — or, ideally, create the deficit with a combination of extra calories burned and fewer calories eaten.

*Another way to look at this:* One pound of fat is simply a storage room for 3,500 calories. However, this number doesn't always hold true in real life. Not every individual will lose exactly one pound by creating a 3,500-calorie deficit. Different people may process calories differently, as indicated by the twins studies described in Question #6. Still, the 3,500-calorie formula is a good general rule.

## Question #31: How do scientists figure out how many calories are burned during any given activity?

*The short answer:* They use one of two methods, direct calorimetry or indirect calorimetry.

### Direct Calorimetry

Direct calorimetry measures the amount of heat (or energy) given off by your body. As we explain in Question #29, a calorie is simply a measure of heat. So if you know how much heat your body produces during a particular activity, you can determine the number of calories you burn while doing that activity.

The downside of direct calorimetry is that it's expensive, complicated, and impractical. It involves a large, airtight chamber and about a thousand more wires and connections than are sticking out the back of your VCR. You need a trained scientist who can decipher an encyclopedia of readouts and mathematical formulas and who knows how to control for factors such as heat given off by the electronic measuring equipment and errors caused by dehydration. All in all, it's not a very practical way to find out how many calories you burn while jogging on the treadmill.

### Indirect Calorimetry

More commonly used, because it's easier and cheaper, is indirect calorimetry, a method of measuring oxygen consumption (also known as VO2, as we explain in Question #128). To determine how many calories you burn while cycling, for example, you sit on a bike while a scientist fits you with a plastic mouth tube. This tube is attached to a contraption known as a metabolic cart, which looks like a cross between an airplane control panel and a hotel room-service cart. As you pedal, you breathe into the tube and the scientist notes the difference between the amount of oxygen in the air you inhale and the air you exhale. Since every liter of oxygen consumed is equivalent to an average of 4.82 calories burned, the measurement of oxygen consumption gives you a reasonably accurate indicator of total calories burned.

Most calorie estimates, including the ones we include in this book, are based on indirect calorimetry. Consider these numbers passable estimates, but keep in mind that, depending on your age, gender, fitness level, and a lot of other factors, your personal caloric expenditure may not exactly match the numbers on a chart.

## Question #32: Which cardio activities burn the most calories?

*The short answer:* Some activities have the potential to burn more calories than others, but they won't do you any good if you flame out in 30 seconds. Any activity that you can perform at a decent intensity for a length of time will ultimately be a good calorie burner for you.

*A 150-pound person* will blaze through nearly 19 calories a minute running at a speed of 10 mph, but not too many of us are capable of sustaining that pace for more than a few minutes without being carried away on a stretcher. On the other hand, a brisk 4 mph walk burns only about 5 calories a minute — not exactly a calorie-burning fiesta, but a pace that most of us can maintain for a good long while.

In general, activities that require you to support your weight as you move, like walking and running, have a higher calorie-burn potential than activities such as cycling, where your weight is supported. That's because it takes energy just to hold your body upright. Still, in reality, the situation is more complicated. The number of calories you burn depends upon how much effort you exert, how skilled you are, how much you weigh, and how long you can last without wearing yourself out.

For instance, you might think that running always burns more calories than walking, but that's not the case. Jogging at a barely-pick-up-your-feet pace burns about 8 calories per minute — the same as walking at a pace that's so speedy that you have to hold yourself back from breaking into a run. And a really fit cyclist who can zip along at 18 miles per hour will burn nearly double that amount.

## Calories Burned During Popular Activities

| Body Weight (pounds) | 120 | 130 | 140 | 150 | 160 | 170 | 180 | 190 | 200 |
|---|---|---|---|---|---|---|---|---|---|
| **Activity** | Calories burned per minute | | | | | | | | |
| Aerobic dance | 5.6 | 5.9 | 6.2 | 6.5 | 6.8 | 7.1 | 7.4 | 7.7 | 8.0 |
| Basketball | 7.4 | 7.8 | 8.2 | 8.6 | 9.0 | 9.4 | 9.8 | 10.2 | 10.6 |
| Bicycling | | | | | | | | | |
| 12 mph | 7.4 | 7.8 | 8.2 | 8.6 | 9.0 | 9.4 | 9.8 | 10.2 | 10.6 |
| 15 mph | 9.3 | 9.8 | 10.3 | 10.8 | 11.3 | 11.8 | 12.3 | 12.8 | 13.3 |
| 18 mph | 11.1 | 11.7 | 12.3 | 12.9 | 13.5 | 14.1 | 14.7 | 15.3 | 15.9 |
| Boxing | 8.4 | 8.9 | 9.4 | 9.9 | 10.4 | 10.9 | 11.4 | 11.9 | 12.4 |
| Circuit weight | 7.0 | 7.4 | 7.8 | 8.2 | 8.6 | 9.0 | 9.4 | 9.8 | 10.2 |
| Downhill skiing | 5.8 | 6.1 | 6.4 | 6.7 | 7.0 | 7.3 | 7.6 | 7.9 | 8.2 |
| Golf (carrying clubs) | 5.1 | 5.4 | 5.7 | 6.0 | 6.3 | 6.6 | 6.9 | 7.2 | 7.5 |
| Inline skating | 7.0 | 7.3 | 7.6 | 7.9 | 8.2 | 8.5 | 8.8 | 9.1 | 9.4 |
| Karate | 8.2 | 8.6 | 9.0 | 9.4 | 9.8 | 10.2 | 10.6 | 11.0 | 11.4 |
| Kayaking | 4.8 | 5.0 | 5.2 | 5.4 | 5.6 | 5.8 | 6.0 | 6.2 | 6.4 |
| Racquetball | 6.5 | 6.9 | 7.3 | 7.7 | 8.1 | 8.5 | 8.9 | 9.3 | 9.7 |
| Rowing machine | 4.2 | 4.4 | 4.6 | 4.8 | 5.0 | 5.2 | 5.4 | 5.6 | 5.8 |
| Running | | | | | | | | | |
| 10-minute mile | 9.3 | 9.8 | 10.3 | 10.8 | 11.3 | 11.8 | 12.3 | 12.8 | 13.3 |
| 8-minute mile | 11.6 | 12.3 | 13.0 | 13.7 | 14.4 | 15.1 | 15.8 | 16.5 | 17.2 |
| Ski machine | 8.7 | 9.2 | 9.7 | 10.2 | 10.7 | 11.2 | 11.7 | 12.2 | 12.7 |
| Swimming (yd/min) | | | | | | | | | |
| Breaststroke | | | | | | | | | |
| 20 | 3.8 | 4.1 | 4.5 | 4.8 | 5.1 | 5.4 | 5.7 | 6.0 | 6.4 |
| 30 | 5.7 | 6.2 | 6.7 | 7.1 | 7.6 | 8.1 | 8.6 | 9.1 | 9.5 |
| 40 | 7.6 | 8.3 | 8.9 | 9.6 | 10.2 | 10.9 | 11.5 | 12.2 | 12.8 |
| Front crawl | | | | | | | | | |
| 25 | 3.8 | 4.1 | 4.5 | 4.8 | 5.1 | 5.4 | 5.7 | 6.0 | 6.4 |
| 35 | 5.9 | 6.4 | 6.8 | 7.3 | 7.8 | 8.3 | 8.8 | 9.2 | 9.7 |
| 50 | 8.5 | 9.2 | 9.9 | 10.6 | 11.3 | 12.0 | 12.8 | 13.5 | 14.2 |
| Tennis | | | | | | | | | |
| Singles | 7.4 | 7.8 | 8.2 | 8.6 | 9.0 | 9.4 | 9.8 | 10.2 | 10.6 |
| Doubles | 6.5 | 6.9 | 7.3 | 7.7 | 8.1 | 8.5 | 8.9 | 9.3 | 9.7 |
| Walking | | | | | | | | | |
| 3 mph, flat | 3.3 | 3.5 | 3.7 | 3.9 | 4.1 | 4.3 | 4.5 | 4.7 | 4.9 |
| 3.5 mph, flat | 3.8 | 4.1 | 4.4 | 4.7 | 5.0 | 5.3 | 5.6 | 5.9 | 6.2 |
| 4 mph, flat | 5.5 | 5.9 | 6.3 | 6.7 | 7.1 | 7.5 | 7.9 | 8.3 | 8.7 |
| 3.5 mph, hill | 5.6 | 5.9 | 6.2 | 6.5 | 6.8 | 7.1 | 7.4 | 7.7 | 8.0 |

So what's the best approach to burning the largest number of calories possible? Choose an activity you can keep up for an entire workout without hurting yourself — and, may we add, one that doesn't bore you to tears. The chart on page 47 gives some rough calorie-burning estimates for popular athletic activities. Keep in mind that your true calorie burn may be dialed up or down depending on your personal and workout variables. Also note that these figures are for the gross — not net — number of calories burned. In other words, they include the approximate number of calories your body burns at rest as well as the extra calories you burn through the exercise.

## Question #33: Which cardio machine burns the most calories?

*The short answer:* If you exercise at the same level of perceived effort on all the machines, you'll likely burn the most calories on the treadmill. But this doesn't mean the treadmill is the best machine for *you*.

*In one study,* researchers from the Medical College of Wisconsin and the Veterans Affairs Medical Center in Milwaukee tested six indoor machines: treadmill, cross-country skiing simulator, rowing machine, stairclimbing machine, stationary bicycle, and stationary bicycle with arm handles. They instructed subjects to exercise on each machine at the same perceived level of effort, such as "hard" or "very hard." The treadmill ranked tops for calories burned (and for aerobic demand on the heart and lungs) while the stationary bike ranked at the bottom, burning about 40 percent fewer calories than the treadmill. Studies that have included the elliptical trainer have found that they're nearly on a par with the treadmill.

However, none of this means you should put your stairclimber or stationary bike up for sale on eBay. If you consider the treadmill a "dreadmill" and prefer climbing or pedaling in place, you're more likely to work harder for longer periods — and thereby burn more calories — on the stairclimber or bike. Any cardio machine can burn a significant number of calories, so use the one you enjoy the most.

Besides, the treadmill does have its minuses. Running has a higher injury rate than lower-impact activities, and most people can't read while they're jogging on the treadmill, a drawback for anyone who relies on *Us Weekly* to get through a cardio workout. Dividing your exercise time among a variety of cardio machines can prevent overuse injuries and help keep you motivated. When you do use the treadmill, be sure that you don't hang on to the front or side railings; otherwise, you'll use a lot less muscle and burn fewer calories.

The chart on pages 52–53 lists the average calorie burn per minute for different machines and body weights. Note that these calorie figures, like those in the chart on page 47, are for the gross — not net — number of calories burned.

## Question #34: Will I burn as many calories running on the treadmill as I do running outdoors?

*The short answer:* If you're running at speeds up to about 9 miles per hour (a 6:40-minute-mile pace), treadmill running burns about the same number of calories as running outdoors. But above 9 mph, treadmill running burns up to 8 percent fewer calories.

*On a treadmill* you don't have to overcome wind resistance — wind currents that you create by pushing through the air at faster speeds. Also, at higher speeds, the belt moving under your feet propels you along to a certain extent. Wind resistance is also the reason that, when running uphill outdoors, you burn one or two calories per minute more for each two degrees of incline than you do when running uphill on a treadmill.

When you walk, either on flat ground or on an incline, you burn the same number of calories on the treadmill as you do outdoors, since you don't move at speeds fast enough to work up any serious wind resistance.

## Question #35: Can I trust the calorie counters on exercise equipment?

*The short answer:* Only to a point. Calorie readouts on gym and home cardio exercise machines typically overestimate the number of calories actually burned by 10 to 30 percent — sometimes by as much as 50 percent. Treadmills tend to be the most accurate because they've been studied the longest and the formulas they use to determine calorie burn are the most well-established.

*If you're planning to stay* on the stairclimber until you burn off every single calorie of last night's Oreo cheesecake, you might want to keep climbing for a good while after you hit your calorie target. That's because the calorie readouts on cardio machines can be wildly unreliable.

Consider: In a study conducted at Appalachian State University in North Carolina, subjects who exercised on five different machines burned an average of 255 calories according to the equipment displays — but only 187 calories according to the sophisticated lab equipment that was monitoring them. That's a difference of about 30 percent. This study is just one of a half dozen recent investigations showing major discrepancies between machine readouts and actual calories burned.

When a machine doesn't ask you to enter your body weight, the inaccuracies tend to be compounded. This usually means the machine has defaulted to information based on a 150-pound exerciser. So if you weigh less, the machine overestimates your burn rate; if you weigh more, the readout will be an underestimate. Also, many machines use formulas that don't take into account additional factors that contribute to calorie burn, such as speed and fitness level. As you become more fit, your body adapts to the challenge of exercise and you burn fewer calories for a given amount of work.

Machine readouts will be even less accurate if you use improper form. For instance, if you drape yourself over the stairclimber console or clutch the front rail of the treadmill like a water-skier, you're making your workout much easier, and the calorie readout may be off by as much as 50 percent.

To increase the accuracy of the calorie information on a machine, it's a good idea to punch in a weight that's about 20 percent lower than your actual weight. (Yes, we're giving you license to lie about your weight!) But even then, don't put too much stock in the number. No exercise machine will give you an exact calorie count unless you go into an exercise lab where scientists can measure your heart rate and the amount of oxygen in your lungs.

## Question #36: Will I burn more calories if I carry hand weights while walking?

*The short answer:* You might burn a few more calories, but the increased risk of injury isn't worth it.

*Carrying hand weights* would seem like an obvious way to boost the number of calories you burn while walking, but we don't recommend this. Walking with weights burns only about 7 to 15 percent more calories — a mere 17 to 36 extra calories over the course of an hour for a 150-pound person walking at a 20-minute-per-mile pace. And at least half the extra calories burned come from exaggerating your arm swing, not from holding the weights.

What's more, those few additional calories come at the cost of a lot of additional strain to your delicate wrist, elbow, and shoulder joints. Each pound of weight you carry shoots ten times the amount of force and stress up your arm. The greatest amount of stress occurs at the top of the arm swing, where your muscles are the least likely to offer any shock absorption to your shoulder and elbow joints.

Waving hand weights around as part of your aerobics routine is not only a bad idea for safety reasons but may actually result in *fewer* calories burned. Any additional calories burned by holding the weights appear to be offset by the need to keep the weights under control as you move your arms and feet. The only way not to clunk yourself on the head with a 2-pounder or take out an en-

## Calories Burned per Minute on Cardio Equipment

| Body Weight (pounds) Activity | 120 | 130 | 140 | 150 | 160 | 170 | 180 | 190 | 200 |
|---|---|---|---|---|---|---|---|---|---|
| **Treadmill** | | | | | | | | | |
| Walking, 3.0 mph | 3.1 | 3.4 | 3.7 | 3.9 | 4.2 | 4.5 | 4.7 | 5.0 | 5.2 |
| Walking, 4.0 mph | 4.2 | 4.6 | 5.0 | 5.3 | 5.7 | 6.0 | 6.4 | 6.7 | 7.1 |
| Walking, 4.5 mph | 4.6 | 5.0 | 5.4 | 5.8 | 6.1 | 6.5 | 6.9 | 7.3 | 7.7 |
| Walking, moderate incline, 3.0 mph | 5.5 | 6.0 | 6.4 | 6.9 | 7.4 | 7.8 | 8.3 | 8.7 | 9.2 |
| Walking, moderate incline, 4.0 mph | 7.0 | 7.6 | 8.2 | 8.8 | 9.4 | 10.0 | 10.6 | 11.1 | 11.7 |
| Walking, moderate incline, 4.5 mph | 7.8 | 8.4 | 9.1 | 9.7 | 10.4 | 11.0 | 11.7 | 12.3 | 13.0 |
| Running, 6.0 mph | 9.7 | 10.5 | 11.3 | 12.2 | 13.0 | 13.8 | 14.6 | 15.4 | 16.2 |
| Running, 7.0 mph | 11.2 | 12.1 | 13.1 | 14.0 | 14.9 | 15.8 | 16.8 | 17.7 | 18.6 |
| Running, 8.0 mph | 12.6 | 13.7 | 14.8 | 15.8 | 16.9 | 17.9 | 19.0 | 20.0 | 21.1 |
| Running, 9.0 mph | 14.1 | 15.3 | 16.5 | 17.6 | 18.8 | 20.0 | 21.2 | 22.3 | 23.5 |
| Running, slight incline, 6.0 mph | 10.9 | 11.8 | 12.7 | 13.6 | 14.5 | 15.5 | 16.4 | 17.3 | 18.2 |
| Running, slight incline, 7.0 mph | 12.6 | 13.6 | 14.7 | 15.7 | 16.8 | 17.8 | 18.9 | 19.9 | 20.9 |
| **Stationary Cycle** | | | | | | | | | |
| Low intensity | 3.8 | 4.1 | 4.4 | 4.7 | 5.0 | 5.3 | 5.6 | 5.9 | 6.2 |
| Medium intensity | 5.6 | 6.0 | 6.4 | 6.8 | 7.2 | 7.6 | 8.0 | 8.4 | 8.8 |
| High intensity | 7.4 | 7.9 | 8.4 | 8.9 | 9.4 | 9.9 | 10.4 | 10.9 | 11.4 |

## Calorie Burned per Minute on Cardio Equipment (continued)

| Body Weight (pounds) | 120 | 130 | 140 | 150 | 160 | 170 | 180 | 190 | 200 |
|---|---|---|---|---|---|---|---|---|---|
| **Activity** | | | | | | | | | |
| **Rower** | | | | | | | | | |
| Low intensity | 4.4 | 4.7 | 5.1 | 5.4 | 5.8 | 6.1 | 6.4 | 6.8 | 7.1 |
| Medium intensity | 6.6 | 7.1 | 7.6 | 8.1 | 8.6 | 9.2 | 9.7 | 10.2 | 10.7 |
| High intensity | 8.0 | 8.5 | 9.0 | 9.5 | 10.0 | 10.5 | 11.0 | 11.5 | 12.0 |
| **Elliptical Trainer** | | | | | | | | | |
| No hill, no resistance | 6.1 | 6.6 | 7.1 | 7.6 | 8.1 | 8.6 | 9.1 | 9.6 | 10.1 |
| Resistance, no hill | 8.1 | 8.7 | 9.4 | 10.1 | 10.8 | 11.4 | 12.1 | 12.8 | 13.5 |
| No resistance, no hill, fast speed | 7.5 | 8.1 | 8.7 | 9.3 | 10.0 | 10.6 | 11.2 | 11.8 | 12.5 |
| Hill incline | 6.4 | 7.0 | 7.5 | 8.0 | 8.6 | 9.1 | 9.7 | 10.2 | 10.7 |
| **Cycle with Arms** | 5.9 | 6.2 | 6.5 | 6.8 | 7.1 | 7.4 | 7.7 | 8.0 | 8.3 |
| **Recumbent Bike** | | | | | | | | | |
| Low intensity | 3.5 | 3.8 | 4.1 | 4.3 | 4.7 | 5.0 | 5.3 | 5.6 | 5.9 |
| Medium intensity | 4.4 | 4.7 | 5.1 | 5.4 | 5.8 | 6.2 | 6.5 | 6.9 | 7.2 |
| High intensity | 5.8 | 6.3 | 6.8 | 7.3 | 7.8 | 8.3 | 8.8 | 9.3 | 9.8 |
| **Stairclimber** | | | | | | | | | |
| Low intensity | 3.9 | 4.2 | 4.5 | 4.8 | 5.1 | 5.4 | 5.7 | 6.0 | 6.3 |
| Medium intensity | 6.9 | 7.3 | 7.7 | 8.1 | 8.5 | 8.9 | 9.3 | 9.7 | 10.1 |
| High intensity | 8.8 | 9.3 | 9.8 | 10.3 | 10.8 | 11.3 | 11.8 | 12.3 | 12.8 |
| **Stairclimber — Stair Simulator** | 6.5 | 6.9 | 7.3 | 7.7 | 8.1 | 8.5 | 8.9 | 9.3 | 9.7 |

tire wall of mirrors is to slow down. And when you slow down, you burn fewer calories.

## Question #37: Will I burn more calories running on the beach than on the street?

*The short answer:* Yes. When you slog through an uneven and variable surface like sand, your muscles have to work harder, so you burn more calories. However, jogging at the beach isn't for everyone.

*Ever watch the lifeguards* on *Baywatch* dash down to the shore, gracefully streaking toward their latest lifesaving mission? They make it look effortless. Well, that's what slow motion is for. If you've ever actually tried to sprint through sand, whether it's the hard, wet stuff near the surf or the dry, grainy sand farther up on the beach, chances are you won't look like Pamela Anderson on TV. Your feet will sink a few centimeters and you'll have to lift your feet higher to pull them out. Your ankles will wobble as they adjust to the uneven terrain. Half the battle is trying to maintain your balance.

All that hard work translates into a higher calorie burn. In fact, studies show that walking on sand burns twice to 2.7 times as many calories as walking on a hard surface at a corresponding speed. Running on sand burns about 1.6 times more calories than running on a harder surface such as dirt, asphalt, or concrete, and you burn more calories on dry sand than wet sand. In terms of calorie burn, it doesn't matter whether you wear shoes or go barefoot.

But before you rush out and join the nearest lifeguard corps, know that the extra calorie burn comes at a price. Because you have to lift your feet up and out of the sand without the benefit of good traction, sand is very hard on the joints, especially the hips, knees, and ankles. Also, as anyone who has ever run on the beach knows, it's very easy to twist an ankle or wrench a knee this way.

If you're prone to joint pain, consider sticking to dirt surfaces or a track. Sand can aggravate tendon and cartilage injuries as well. If you just can't resist a run on the beach, wear your running shoes for the extra support and cushioning and stay near the firmer, more stable wet pack near the shoreline.

## Question #38: I hear jumping rope is one of the best ways to burn calories. Just how effective is it?

*The short answer:* You burn between 8 and 19 calories per minute, depending on how much you weigh and how fast you spin the rope.

*Since you have to support* your body weight while you jump (as opposed to resting some of your weight on, say, the seat of a bike), the heavier you are, the more calories you burn for a given amount of jumping. Also, the faster you turn the rope, the more muscle is required to power the rope and propel you upward off the floor, thereby increasing your calorie burn.

### Calories Burned While Jumping Rope

| Weight | | | | | Turns/minute | | | | | |
|---|---|---|---|---|---|---|---|---|---|---|
| (lbs) | 110 | 120 | 130 | 140 | 150 | 160 | 170 | 180 | 190 | 200 |
| 70 | 8.5 | 9.0 | 10.0 | 11.1 | 11.6 | 12.6 | 13.1 | 14.1 | 15.1 | 15.6 |
| 110 | 9.3 | 9.9 | 11.0 | 12.1 | 12.6 | 13.8 | 14.3 | 15.4 | 16.0 | 16.5 |
| 130 | 10.3 | 10.9 | 12.8 | 13.4 | 14.7 | 15.3 | 15.9 | 17.1 | 17.8 | 18.4 |
| 145 | 10.4 | 11.0 | 13.5 | 14.2 | 14.8 | 15.4 | 16.0 | 17.3 | 18.5 | 19.2 |

## Question #39: Will I burn more calories exercising in hot or cold weather?

*The short answer:* You burn about the same number of calories regardless of the weather, unless you're so cold that you start to shiver.

*Shivering is an involuntary clenching* of muscles; its purpose is to generate heat and warm you up. When your teeth are chattering and every muscle in your body is tight and tense, you burn nearly four times more calories than usual. And when it's so cold that in addition to shivering, you have to hop from foot to foot and rub your hands together to keep warm, you burn up to 400 additional calories per hour.

But this isn't a good reason to go out jogging in January in North Dakota wearing nothing but shorts and a tank top. Sure, you'll burn more calories than if you work out properly clothed or indoors on the treadmill, but you'll also risk hypothermia and frostbite.

You don't burn any extra calories by sweating it up in one of those yoga classes where they crank the temperature to 100 degrees, either. It may seem like you're melting away pounds more quickly, but in reality you're just shedding more water than usual. As soon as you take a drink, you replace the water weight. And if you don't drink up, you risk dehydration.

## Question #40: Will I burn more calories on a stairclimbing machine or climbing real steps?

*The short answer:* You'll probably burn more calories climbing actual stairs, but there are trade-offs.

*Walking up the staircase* in your office building burns about 10 calories per minute for a 150-pound person. Pick up the pace to a sprint and you'll burn an impressive 18 calories per minute — if your knees don't buckle and you don't poop out by the time you hit the third flight. On a stairclimbing machine — the kind that involves pressing on two foot plates — exercising at a moderate intensity burns about 8 calories per minute provided you don't cheat; white-knuckling the handrails or draping yourself over the console can cut your calorie burn in half.

Why the big difference? With actual steps, you use more muscle — to pick up your feet, bend your hip and knee to lift your leg, and shift your weight onto your front leg. But on machines like the StairMaster, you simply shift your weight from foot to foot. Not that this is necessarily a breeze; depending on the intensity level you program in, keeping up with the machine can be plenty tough, and you can burn as many as 10 calories per minute if you use good form.

Even though actual stairclimbing burns more calories than virtual stairclimbing, it's not necessarily a better choice for exercise. Climbing real steps places a lot of stress on your joints, especially your knees, ankles, and lower back. Plus, with virtual stairs, what goes up does *not* come down. Descending steps burns only about 4 calories per minute and places more pressure on the front of the kneecap than going up. However, none of this should stop you from climbing up and down steps you encounter during the course of your daily life. Climbing steps is a great way to burn calories and isn't likely to bother your joints unless they're already shot to begin with.

There's one type of stair workout that, to a large extent, offers the best of both worlds: rolling staircase machines. These look something like short escalators, except *you* have to do the work. If you don't climb the steps fast enough, you'll stumble and slide off the machine. On these contraptions (the most popular brand is the Stepmill, formerly called the Gauntlet), you burn as many calories as you do on real steps, assuming you don't clutch the side rails, but you never have to descend. Just keep in mind that these machines offer a higher-impact workout than stairclimbers.

## Question #41: What does *metabolism* actually mean?

*The short answer:* Your metabolism is the rate at which your body uses energy — burns calories — at any given moment, whether you're watching *Law & Order* or sprinting on the treadmill. However, when people use the term *metabolism* in conversation — as in "I have such a slow metabolism!" — they're typically referring to *resting* metabolism, the calorie burn required to keep your body alive and humming.

*Even when you're sound asleep,* your body uses energy to keep your heart beating, your kidneys functioning, your skin cells regenerating, and so on. Typically, your resting metabolism accounts for 60 to 75 percent of your total calorie burn for the day. (Your activity level accounts for another 15 to 30 percent, depending on how much you move around. The calorie burn associated with eating and digesting food accounts for about 5 or 10 percent of your total daily energy expenditure.) Resting metabolism, also known as "resting metabolic rate," varies quite a lot between individuals, depending primarily on body size, genetics, and muscle mass.

There are dozens of methods for estimating metabolism. Some research labs are outfitted with large, airtight rooms in which subjects can eat, sleep, and exercise; air is drawn into and out of the chamber, and measurements of oxygen and carbon dioxide are used to determine metabolism. Without going to all that trouble, you can get a reasonable estimate by having a trainer or registered dietitian measure your calorie-burn rate on a hand-held device like the Body Gem (available through healthetech.com). You breathe into a mouthpiece for 10 to 15 minutes while the Body Gem calculates the difference between the percentage of oxygen in the air you breathe in versus the percentage in the air you exhale. This number correlates with the number of calories you burn per minute, allowing you to estimate your resting metabolism over 24 hours. This type of testing is being offered at many gyms and hospitals across the country.

## Question #42: Will regular cardio exercise boost my resting metabolism?

*The short answer:* No.

*Some studies show that people* who do cardiovascular exercise regularly have speedier resting metabolisms than sedentary people. But this is likely due to a small carryover effect from their last workout — the so-called "afterburn" described in Question #44 —

rather than some permanent change in metabolism. In studies where researchers have waited to measure resting metabolism until several days after regular exercisers' last workouts, no increase has been detected. If you do cardio exercise regularly, you'll get a temporary metabolism boost after each workout, but just know that it's an advantage that won't last if you stop exercising.

## Question #43: Can weight training rev up my metabolism?

*The short answer:* Yes, but not as much as some fitness magazines and trainers would have you believe. Still, regular weight training can offset much, if not most, of the muscle loss and metabolism decline that typically comes with age or dieting, thereby helping to stave off extra pounds.

*"Mega Metabolism Boost!"* "The Metabolism Jump-Start Workout!" "Burn Extra Calories 24 Hours a Day, Even as You Sleep!" Glance at the latest fitness magazine covers and you might get the impression that weight training will make your metabolism go from 0 to 60 faster than a Lamborghini. Well, the reality isn't quite so sensational.

It's true that lifting weights builds muscle, and the more muscle you have, the more calories your body will burn at rest. But what the magazines don't mention is that it takes a lot of extra muscle to dramatically rev up your resting metabolic rate. Although you may have heard that you burn an extra 50 or 100 calories per day for each pound of muscle you build, that figure is not supported by science, says metabolism researcher Christopher Melby, Dr.P.H., head of the Metabolic Fitness Laboratory at Colorado State University in Fort Collins. "It's actually closer to 10 to 15 calories, so you really can't expect to see much of an increase in metabolic rate with the typical 3- to 4-pound increase in muscle mass."

It's actually unclear what you *can* expect to see. Weight-training studies have produced radically different findings, some showing an increase in fat-free mass of up to 4 pounds over 12 to 16 weeks, along with a boost in resting metabolism of up to 10 percent, or 160 calories a day. But other studies — the ones that don't make the headlines — show no increase at all in resting metabolism over three to four months, even despite increases in fat-free mass. Still other studies show a slight increase in metabolism despite no increase in fat-free mass, and some studies show no detectible increases in fat-free mass or metabolism. What's going on?

For one thing, most studies last just three to four months, which isn't enough time for many people to build enough muscle to cause a significant metabolism spike. In many cases, the increase may be so small as to be within the margin of error for measurement. Also fat-free mass isn't the same thing as muscle; increases in fat-free mass may, in part, reflect increases in water content, not muscle. The fact that research results have differed so greatly suggests that the issue isn't cut-and-dried.

You're most likely to get a dramatic metabolism boost if you lift weights for several years, gaining more than the typical few pounds of muscle. And over the long haul, even an extra 40 calories burned a day could make a difference in weight control. But here's an important caveat: Even if you do get a metabolism boost from packing on muscle, you can't rest on your laurels — or, in this case, on your butt. In some research, a metabolic boost proved to be irrelevant because subjects became less active during the rest of the day. Even though their resting metabolic rates increased, the total number of daily calories they burned did not. So just make sure you don't tell yourself, "Hey, I did my workout, now I can surf the Net for hours on end."

None of this means you should put down your barbells. Quite the contrary. Lifting weights is the key to preserving your muscle mass and metabolism as you get older. Sedentary people tend to lose at least one-third of their muscle from age 30 to age 70, but consistent weightlifting probably can offset most of the decline. With more muscle and a higher resting metabolic rate, you're less likely to gain fat. Lifting weights also can offset — by nearly half — the muscle loss experienced by dieters.

### Question #44: Is it true that my metabolism stays elevated after a workout?

*The short answer:* Yes, and the harder you exercise, the greater your "afterburn" will be. Weight training gives you more of a calorie-burn bonus than moderate aerobic exercise, but for the average person, the afterburn may not amount to all that much for either type of workout.

*Afterburn is an appealing concept:* For all the effort you expend during a workout, you burn additional calories afterward without even trying — sort of like a buy-3-get-1-free deal at the store. However, how many "free" calories you get depends on how long — and, to a greater extent, how hard — you work out.

You're likely to get the greatest afterburn from a long, hard weight-training workout. In one study, fit men who completed a killer, 90-minute strength workout, performing 60 sets with little rest, experienced an 11 percent metabolism increase two hours after the workout. The next morning, 15 hours after the workout, their metabolisms were still elevated by a hefty 9 percent, which would translate into about 150 extra calories burned. While the numbers are impressive, the workouts were far longer and more strenuous than most people have the time, fitness, and motivation to maintain. For a more typical workout — say, three sets of ten exercises — researchers guess the afterburn might last only a few hours and add up to no more than 50 to 75 calories, if that.

Still, that's a decent bang for your buck, and it's a considerably greater bonus than most people are likely to get from the afterburn of a cardio workout. "For the amount of exercise most people do — about 30 to 45 minutes — the afterburn is going to be less than 30 calories," says Christopher Melby. Although any extra boost is nice, keep in mind that the number of calories you burn after a cardio workout is a small fraction of what you burn while you exercise.

Why does weight training produce a greater afterburn than cardio exercise? In addition to being a more intense type of workout, lifting weights seems to elevate hormones, such as epinephrine, that simulate metabolic rate. It's also possible that the microscopic tissue damage caused by weightlifting may compel the body to expend extra energy for tissue repair.

## Question #45: If I had anorexia, is my metabolism permanently damaged?

*The short answer:* Not usually. It may be damaged in the short run, but eventually your metabolism should return to normal.

*People who've had anorexia nervosa* tend to lose a lot of muscle mass, which results in a sluggish metabolism. The body perceives that it's being starved and compensates by burning fewer calories.

Those who fully recover from this eating disorder often complain that their metabolism remains slow even though they have resumed sensible eating and exercise habits. A study reported in the *European Journal of Eating Disorders* gives some credence to this idea, at least during the initial phases of recovery. Researchers from several Italian universities used skinfold calipers (defined in Question #10) to measure the body-fat percentage of ten women who had made a full recovery from anorexia and had maintained a stabilized, normal weight for at least five months. The results: Up to 76 percent of the weight gained was fat — a much higher percentage than a typical dieter's fat regain — and their abdominal and biceps skinfolds were significantly thicker than those of subjects who'd never suffered from anorexia. The recovered anorexics averaged about 8 percent less fat-free mass than control subjects. The researchers concluded that recovered anorexics appear to preferentially regain fat, especially in the abdominal, arm, and hip regions, and that their body composition does not completely normalize after they gain weight.

However, many long-term studies seem to indicate that a slow metabolism and abnormal fat storage may ultimately be reversible.

It may take a year, or even longer, but normal fat and muscle distribution can come back with nutritious eating and regular exercise. Weight training, especially, can help build muscle.

## Question #46: Can hot peppers speed up my metabolism?

*The short answer:* Not to any degree that will help you lose weight.

*When you eat something so spicy* that you break out in a sweat, your skin gets tingly, and you feel like smoke is emanating from your ears, your metabolic rate jumps up briefly. But there's no reason to believe that munching on hot peppers will ever take the place of a cardio kickboxing class or a brisk walk. Peppers simply don't give you a metabolic boost that's significant enough or long-lasting enough to help you lose an ounce.

There have been a few highly publicized studies hypothesizing that the chemical capsaicin, which makes peppers and some other spicy foods hot, may act as an appetite suppressant. However, the effect appears to be temporary, and in some studies, when the subjects ate less after partaking of a hot-pepper appetizer, they made up for it by eating more at subsequent meals.

# Weight Loss: Strategies, Supplements, Drugs, and Surgery

Although most of us keep regaining the weight we lose, we're eternally optimistic — eager to try the latest diet plan, workout contraption, metabolism pill, prescription fat-blocker. When one approach doesn't pan out, we move on to the next, sometimes before even receiving the Visa bill for the last one. Score one for the weight-loss industry.

In fact, it's hard to think of any other industry where so much money — more than $30 billion spent by consumers each year — is spent on products that consistently fail to deliver what they promise. Yet consumers often blame themselves when the scale doesn't budge. Have you ever followed a new weight-loss plan, failed to get results, and wondered: What did I do wrong?

In many cases, the mistake was purchasing the supplement, device, or program in the first place — falling prey to advertising hype. Or perhaps, if no products were involved, the problem was simply having unrealistic expectations, putting faith in an approach that simply defies the fundamental principles of weight loss.

In this section, we explain which strategies actually work (yes, it's possible to lose weight and keep it off for good) and which are destined to fail — and may even be harmful to your health. We answer your questions about weight-loss drugs and supplements, revealing loopholes that allow for misleading labels. We also cover surgical procedures such as liposuction and stomach stapling, explaining who's a good candidate for these procedures and what the success rates are. And if you've ever wondered how sumo wrestlers get so hefty, whether yo-yo dieting makes you fatter, or whether you're likely to gain weight after you get married, all that is here, too.

## Question #47: If I need to lose weight in a hurry, what's the best strategy?

*The short answer:* Sorry, there isn't one! Losing weight in a hurry is a bad idea.

*Type "quick weight loss"* into any Internet search engine and you'll hit on thousands of get-thin-quick schemes, but the cold, hard truth is that they're all going to backfire. Any diet that drastically cuts your calorie intake — whether it's the cabbage diet, the grapefruit diet, the Hollywood diet, or the chocolate-fudge diet — can take pounds off quickly. But you're going to put those pounds right back on if you make radical changes that you can't sustain. Besides, much of the weight you lose right away is water, not fat, and when you go on a crash diet you're likely to lose more muscle tissue than when you shed pounds at a slower rate.

You can also forget about those soaps that claim to wash away cellulite, as well as slim patches, fat-burning pills, and fat-melting devices. Like gimmicky diets, they won't help you lose weight or keep it off. The only thing they're likely to lighten up is your wallet.

Above all, losing weight quickly isn't good for your health. It can seriously compromise your intake of essential nutrients, and some rapid weight-loss plans can leave you dangerously weak and dehydrated.

Chances are you didn't gain those extra 30 pounds in a few weeks; you can't expect to lose them in two weeks' time for your 20th high school reunion or Caribbean cruise. You're best off aiming to lose ½ to 1 pound a week, perhaps slightly more if you're seriously overweight.

## Question #48: Which is more important for weight loss, diet or exercise?

*The short answer:* Diet probably contributes more to weight loss for most people because it's easier to cut calories than it is to burn them off through exercise. But combining diet and exercise is better for weight control than either strategy alone, and exercise is crucial for keeping the pounds off in the long run.

*A number of studies* have concluded that restricting calories is a better way to drop a pants size than spending more time in the gym. For example, one 12-week trial found that men and women who exercised but did not diet lost .3 percent of their initial body weight while those who dieted but did not exercise lost 8.4 percent of their weight.

But before you toss out your running shoes, consider this important fact: This study, like many others, did not compare diet and exercise on an equal footing. The women in the diet-only group cut 945 calories per day, and the men cut 1,705 calories. Meanwhile, the exercise-only groups walked or jogged for 30 minutes five times a week, expending an average of 255 and 190 calories per session for men and women, respectively. So in this case, comparing diet and exercise is like comparing apples and oranges. When researchers compare subjects who eat 500 fewer calories per day with subjects who burn an extra 500 calories by walking, both groups tend to lose the same amount of weight.

Of course, it takes an hour or more for most of us to burn off 500 calories through exercise but barely a moment to suck down a 500-calorie mocha malt Frappuccino. That's why once you step outside the laboratory, dieting probably plays a bigger role in weight loss than exercise.

Still, it's clear that combining diet and exercise achieves better results than doing either separately. In a review of more than a dozen studies lasting up to a year, the National Institutes of Health found that groups that did aerobic exercise and cut calories lost an average of 4.2 pounds more than groups that just dieted. Groups that added weight training to the mix were rewarded with 2 additional pounds of weight loss on average. And over the long run, research shows, exercise is the single best predictor of who succeeds in keeping off the weight they've lost.

## Question #49: If I lose weight, what are the chances I'll keep it off?

*The short answer:* Although most people — perhaps 95 percent of all dieters — who lose weight regain most or all of it within three years, there are plenty of people who defy the odds. Anyone who sheds pounds slowly and sticks with an exercise program stands a good chance of keeping the weight off.

*Considering that 64 percent of Americans* are overweight or obese and the weight-loss industry isn't exactly in a recession, it's safe to say that most people who lose weight gain most or all of it back. According to obesity researchers and countless surveys of dieters, the number may be 95 percent or greater — and this includes people who lose weight through diet, exercise, or a combination of both.

It's no great mystery why people regain the weight they've worked so hard to lose: They retreat to their old habits, blowing off workouts and nestling back into the recliner. The more complex question is: Why is it so darned hard to stick to the eating and exercise habits that enable people to lose weight in the first place? One reason is that people go to extremes, drastically cutting calories or going bonkers with a new exercise program, rather than making modest lifestyle changes that they can maintain over the long haul. If you've been subsisting for a decade on burgers and fries and then suddenly switch to spinach and tofu, chances are you're going to feel deprived and hungry and fall off the wagon quickly.

Of course, making gradual changes is easier said than done, and it goes against the human instinct for instant gratification. To increase your chances of success, many experts recommend losing no more than ½ pound to 1 pound per week. You can healthfully lose as much as 2 pounds a week, but for many people, especially those who are only slightly overweight, a more modest weekly goal is more realistic. Many people lose considerably more than 2 pounds a week at first, but much of it is water weight. Eventually the weight loss slows down to 1 pound or less a week, and at some point you're bound to hit a plateau.

Although regaining weight is the norm, it is by no means inevitable. Consider the National Weight Control Registry, a collaborative venture between the University of Colorado and the University of Pittsburgh, which keeps tabs on more than 3,000 people who have lost at least 30 pounds and have maintained that loss for at least a year. The average registrant has lost about 60 pounds and has maintained this loss for about five years — no small feat for a group of people who, in two-thirds of the cases, were overweight since childhood.

What's their secret? It's not that they follow a particular diet; in fact, at least half report following no program at all, instead making their own commonsense choices. However, there are two common denominators among the registry participants: exercising regularly and cutting calories. Registry participants report burning about 2,800 calories per week through exercise (about 7 to 11 hours a week, depending on their weight and intensity level) and reducing their calorie intake, primarily by practicing portion control rather than forgoing entire food groups, popping pills, or going on liquid diets.

One particularly interesting finding from the registry participants: The risk of relapse appears to decrease over time. In other words, the longer you keep up with lifestyle changes, the more likely they are to remain a permanent part of your life.

## How They Kept the Weight Off

What are the keys to successful, long-term weight loss? Here's a summary of the exercise and eating habits of participants in the National Weight Control Registry. True, this group represents a minuscule portion of dieters, but the registry does offer some insight into the habits common among people who are successful at weight loss.

- 89 percent changed both their eating habits and physical activity patterns.
- 96 percent exercised regularly, burning on average 2,800 calories a week.

- Fewer than 5 percent followed diets such as the Zone, Sugar Busters!, and Atkins.
- 50 percent ate the same foods they had always eaten but restricted portion size.
- 50 percent counted calories, averaging 1,400 calories per day, spread among five meals.

## Question #50: What's the best way to reduce a paunchy middle?

*The short answer:* You can't target your midsection — or any other area of your body — for weight loss, but research does suggest that cardiovascular exercise is especially effective for reducing abdominal fat.

*You simply cannot make fat disappear* from any area of your body by targeting it with exercise. Nor can you do it by zapping the area with electrical stimulation, rubbing cream onto it, covering it with a patch, or taking a pill "specially designed to reduce your spare tire." But that doesn't stop unscrupulous infomercials from trying to sell a whole host of devices that supposedly have the power to whittle your middle. This fact also does not stop many people from buying these products or believing that crunches and other ab exercises are a good way to melt away abdominal fat.

In reality, your body is predisposed to lose and gain weight in a genetically predetermined pattern, which is different for every individual. You can't change this pattern, but you can lose weight all over your body by eating fewer calories than you burn off. When you lose weight, some of it will come off your middle. This is especially true, research suggests, if you engage in cardio exercise as part of your weight-loss program. In a study published in the *Journal of the American Medical Association,* women who either walked or cycled for 45 minutes five days a week for one year lost 4 percent of their total body fat — and 7 percent of their intra-abdominal fat. More research is needed to determine whether dieting would help reduce abdominal fat even further.

So does that mean exercising your middle is a waste of time? Most definitely not. The ab exercises we describe in Question #166 do a great job of strengthening and toning the muscles that reside underneath your abdominal fat. Stronger ab muscles also help you stand up straighter, and better posture makes your stomach look smaller even if you don't lose an ounce of fat.

## Question #51: What's the best way to slim down saddlebags?

*The short answer:* Fat in the hip and thigh area can be especially stubborn, and there's no way to melt fat off that area specifically. Still, when you lose weight overall — by burning off more calories than you eat — some of it is bound to come off the saddlebags.

*It's a genetic fait accompli:* For those with two X chromosomes, outer-thigh adipose — not so affectionately nicknamed "saddlebags" — tends to get stored disproportionately in the hip and thigh area. And research shows that fat in this area usually clings more stubbornly to the body than fat stored elsewhere.

You can't target your thighs for fat loss, but you can tone this area with weight-training exercises. A regular lifting program that includes exercises such as squats, lunges, and side leg lifts strengthens and firms your hip and thigh muscles and can help reshape the saddlebag area to a certain extent, even if the fat remains. You can also make your saddlebags appear smaller by developing your upper-body muscles. When you widen your shoulders and back, you bring your entire physique into better proportion.

Even if you're not enamored of your saddlebags, at least take comfort in the fact that, unlike fat in the abdominal area, hip and thigh fat is not harmful to your health and may even offer some protection against cardiovascular disease, as we explained in Question #13.

## Question #52: Will yo-yo dieting make me fatter?

*The short answer:* Maybe. Plus, it could be bad for your health.

*"Hey, I can lose ten pounds* — I've done it a hundred times." That seems to be the mantra of the typical American dieter. Repeatedly losing and regaining weight is a common frustration, and research suggests that this pattern may indeed make it progressively harder for people to lose weight. Studies show that people lose weight more slowly on their second attempt than they do on their first.

In the 1980s, when scientists first began researching weight cycling, better known as yo-yo dieting, they speculated that this pattern would make weight loss tougher by causing a metabolism slowdown. The theory seemed sound enough: When dieters lose weight, they lose (in addition to fat) large amounts of muscle, but when they regain weight, researchers guessed, they primarily put on fat. So, the repeated cycle of losing muscle — which burns more calories than fat — and gaining fat would only slow down a dieter's metabolism, making weight loss that much more difficult.

Logical as this theory sounds, research ultimately disproved it. In 1994, the National Institutes of Health and the National Task Force on the Prevention and Treatment of Obesity released a joint statement on weight cycling based on a review of several dozen weight-loss studies. Their conclusion: Yo-yo dieting doesn't seem to cause a long-term metabolic slowdown. As it turns out, even though about 25 percent of weight lost from dieting without exercise is lean body tissue, about 25 percent of regained weight is also lean body mass, including muscle, which builds up to support the extra weight you've gained.

Still, dieters have long complained that they have a tougher time losing weight with each successive attempt, and there is solid research to back them up. Some experts speculate that this type of dieting pattern increases your number of fat cells. Another factor may be age: Every time you try to lose weight, you are, of course, older than you were the last time. As you age, you tend to lose muscle, which slows your metabolism. You may also experience hormonal changes that tend to encourage fat gain. In addition, as people get older, they tend to be less active, which makes weight loss even harder.

Weight-control issues aside, there's another reason for avoiding a constant up-and-down weight pattern: It's rough on the old bod. Weight cycling has been linked to everything from high blood pressure to lower HDL cholesterol levels to heart disease to renal and breast cancer.

## Question #53: Is it better for weight loss if I do short workouts at a fast pace or long workouts at a slow pace?

*The short answer:* The best workout for weight loss is the one that burns the most calories. Period.

*The treadmill at your gym* probably has a slow-paced "fat-burning" program. And the stationary bike probably has a heart-rate chart on its display that recommends a range of heart rates best for weight loss and fat burning. Ignore these. They're vestiges of an outdated belief that long, slow workouts are always better for weight loss than faster, shorter workouts.

This mistaken belief stems from an actual truth: When you burn calories at slower speeds, your body's primary fuel source is fat, whereas at higher intensities, you use primarily the carbohydrate circulating in your bloodstream or stored in your muscle. Misguided exercisers sometimes reason that using higher percentages of fat as fuel must translate into quicker fat loss. But the truth is, the more calories you burn, the closer you inch toward your weight-loss goals, regardless of what type of fuel your body uses for energy.

So does this mean that if your goal is weight loss, you should set your treadmill on warp factor 6 every single workout? Of course not. Too much high-intensity exercise can leave you burned-out, sore, or prone to injuries. You're better off striking a balance between high- and low-intensity workouts over the course of each week. And certainly, there are a lot of workouts that fall somewhere between a leisurely walk and a killer sprint.

## Question #54: Can walking help me lose weight?

*The short answer:* Absolutely — if you do enough of it and watch what you eat as well.

*While it's true that walking* doesn't burn calories as quickly as jogging or Spinning or other high-intensity workouts (see Questions #32 and 33 for calorie info), scores of studies have shown it to be a very effective weight-loss tool. For example, a study published in the *Journal of the American Medical Association* found that brisk walking is effective for reducing deep abdominal fat, the most dangerous kind of fat. And a University of Colorado study found that if people could commit to walking 2,000 steps a day more than they do now — the equivalent of about one mile or about 15 minutes' worth of movement — they may not necessarily lose weight but would probably stop gaining. The typical adult gains about one pound a year, which means we're eating, on average, an excess of 10 to 30 calories a day. The 100 calories per day burned off from walking 2,000 steps would more than compensate for this excess.

Researchers have also found that walking an additional 6,000 steps a day (or about 3 miles) is the point at which the pounds really start coming off, as long as it is done in conjunction with sensible eating habits such as portion control. A report from the Institute of Medicine of the National Academies makes similar recommendations, advising one hour of daily walking or other moderate exercise for weight loss. What's more, the majority of participants in the National Weight Control Registry, an ongoing survey of long-term weight-loss success stories (see Question #49), report walking as one of their major weight-loss strategies.

So if walking doesn't exactly turn your body into a calorie-burning inferno, why does it seem to work so well? For one thing, walking has a major advantage over most other fitness activities: It doesn't require any stuff. No helmets, gloves, wrenches, pumps, kneepads, wrist guards, caps, goggles, pools, or poles. Just lace up your shoes, open the front door, and you're off. Plus, unless you're a toddler, walking has virtually no learning curve.

Of course, running is equally accessible and convenient, but it also has a much higher injury rate. Walking is considerably easier on your joints, tendons, and ligaments (although a small percentage of walkers do get injured from overdoing it or wearing the wrong shoes). Walking is also less exhausting, so you may be more likely to stick to your program. Running may burn twice the calories per minute as walking, but if you quit after five minutes because your knees feel like they're about to explode, what's the point?

Walking is also an especially good weight-loss activity because it's so easily adaptable to your fitness level. As you become more fit, you can walk faster, walk more often, walk up steeper hills, or walk for longer periods.

## Question #55: I've heard that swimming isn't as effective for weight loss as other forms of exercise. Is this true?

*The short answer:* Swimming can probably help you lose weight, but for the average person, it may not work as well as other aerobic activities.

*As a workout,* swimming has an uneven reputation. Although it gets high marks for being easy on your body and improving cardiovascular fitness, some research shows that, for recreational swimming, it's less effective for weight loss than land-based workouts.

What's going on? Does the cold water somehow reduce fat burning? Does swimming stimulate the appetite? Theories abound.

On the recreational level, this much is clear: Most people can't swim fast enough or long enough to burn significant numbers of calories. Swimming requires considerably more skill than walking or cycling, and most of us don't have the technique to glide through the water at high speeds. Fit, fish-like swimmers may burn 600 calories or considerably more in an hour workout; an unskilled swimmer may flop across the pool at only half the speed and tire out after 20 minutes, burning just 100 calories.

Still, calorie burning may not entirely explain the conundrum, since elite swimmers burn just as many calories as elite runners, yet have, on average, more body fat than competitive runners. One theory is swimming makes people hungrier, so they eat more. But this notion was refuted by a study that let runners and swimmers eat to their hearts' content in the two hours after a workout; the groups reported the same level of hunger and ate roughly the same number of calories.

In one study, competitive swimmers who swam the longest distances had the least amount of body fat, so swimming does seem to help with weight control. Still, competitive swimmers do tend to have more body fat than competitive runners, despite their mega-yardage workouts. In part this may be due to self-selection. It takes a small, light body to be a good distance runner, so people with that body type may gravitate toward running. In the pool, people with more body fat can succeed and in some cases may perform better than slimmer athletes, especially in endurance events. Swimming marvel Lynne Cox, who has broken records for swimming across the English Channel and other daunting distances, weighs 180 pounds, at 5-foot-6.

If you enjoy swimming and want to lose weight, aim to improve your technique by taking a few lessons or joining a masters program (go to the U.S. Masters Swimming Web site, usms.org, to find a club near you). If you're already a skilled swimmer and still not getting the weight-loss results you'd hoped for, try mixing land-based activities into your workout program.

## Question #56: Does menopause cause women to gain weight?

*The short answer:* Menopause probably does trigger changes that make women more susceptible to weight gain, especially deep in the abdomen, but at this point scientists have more questions than answers.

*This much is clear:* After menopause, which typically occurs around age 50, women burn fewer calories at rest and during exercise, lose muscle at a faster rate, and accumulate more fat deep in the belly. But are these changes due to menopause itself or simply the aging process — or that women are typically less active as they get older?

One study that tried to sort this out followed 35 sedentary premenopausal women ages 44 to 48 for six years. By the end of the study, the women who'd stopped menstruating had lost, on average, 6.6 pounds of fat-free mass, compared with only about 1 pound for the women who remained premenopausal. Their resting metabolisms dropped by about 100 calories per day, compared with just 8 calories for the other group. The menopausal women reported being less physically active to the tune of 127 fewer calories per day, compared with 64 calories for the comparison group. So it's not surprising that the group that went through menopause gained 5.5 pounds of body fat, compared with about 2.2 pounds for the premenopausal women.

Researchers suspect that menopause-related decline in estrogen makes fat cells more likely to store fat and perhaps less likely to release it, but they are still exploring how and why this happens. It's also possible that hormonal changes during menopause stimulate appetite, although this theory hasn't been confirmed in humans. Studies show that rats that lose estrogen eat 10 percent to 20 percent more calories than they need.

Since plenty of evidence shows that menopause-related weight gain is focused deep in the abdominal area, and abdominal fat is strongly linked to risk for diabetes, heart disease, and high blood pressure, experts recommend that women make a concerted effort to stay active as they go through menopause.

## Question #57: Will I gain weight if I quit smoking?

*The short answer:* Maybe. About 80 percent of people who quit smoking see the scale creep up, commonly by 5 to 10 pounds. The other 20 percent either maintain their weight or lose a small amount of weight.

*Among ex-smokers* who do put on pounds, research suggests, the weight gain tends to subside — or even start to reverse itself — after six months to a year. And while former smokers may not lose all of the weight they initially gained, ultimately they are likely to settle at the weight level of people who never smoked. "A lot of smokers are artificially under their ideal body weight, so when they quit, they end up back at what a normal body weight would be," says Douglas Jorenby, Ph.D., an associate professor of medicine at the University of Wisconsin Medical School and director of clinical services at the school's Center for Tobacco Research and Intervention. Studies suggest that nicotine gum and bupropion, an antidepressant shown to help with smoking cessation, may delay weight gain, but as soon as people quit using these aids, they typically experience the same weight gain as people who don't use them.

Why do so many people gain weight after kicking the habit? One reason is that they eat more. When you quit smoking, your senses of taste and smell blossom, so those cinnamon rolls and bacon-and-eggs breakfast platters may suddenly seem more appealing. Women in particular may find themselves craving sweets, some research shows. Common withdrawal symptoms — anxiety, nervousness, and irritability — may also cause ex-smokers to raid the refrigerator. And some turn to food as a way to keep their hands and mouth busy in the absence of cigarettes.

But increased calorie consumption doesn't appear to account for all of the weight gain that ex-smokers experience; the absence of nicotine also seems to play a role. Some studies suggest that nicotine lowers the body's "set-point," the weight at which it intrinsically wants to settle. This may explain why smokers tend to weigh less than nonsmokers, even though they don't eat significantly fewer calories and tend to be more sedentary. "As nicotine clears their system, their set-point goes back to normal," Jorenby says. "Their basal metabolism slows down, and their bodies want to store more fat."

Regular exercise, even 30 minutes a day, can help minimize weight gain after you quit smoking. So can eating more slowly.

Many smokers hurry through dinner so they can smoke; when they quit, they're still in the habit of speed eating, increasing the odds that they'll go back for seconds. Just don't go overboard with exercise and cutting calories. People who start strict diet and exercise programs at the same time they try to quit smoking tend to fail at all the changes.

Even if you do gain some weight after kicking the habit, remember that the dangers of continued smoking far outweigh the risks of putting on a few extra pounds. In fact, some experts estimate that it would take a weight gain of nearly 80 pounds to offset the health benefits that an average smoker gains by quitting.

### Question #58: I've noticed that a lot of people gain weight after they get married. Is there any correlation?

*The short answer:* Probably, although the patterns may be different for men and women.

*If you've ever looked at your wedding picture* and thought, "Yeesh, no way could we fit into *that* gown and tux anymore," you apparently have plenty of company. Women tend to gain weight in the few years following marriage, research suggests, although it's not clear whether the extra pounds are related to couplehood itself or are simply a reflection of the usual tendency to put on pounds with age and having kids. (See Question #238 for information about post-pregnancy weight gain.) The typical man's waistband does not seem to expand immediately after tying the knot, but on average married men are heavier than single or divorced men of the same age, so it may just take longer after getting married for men to gain weight.

Just how many pounds do married people tend to gain after walking down the aisle, and how quickly does the weight pile on? Researchers can't say with certainty. Studies have produced very mixed results — with some showing weight gain for both men and women and others showing weight gain for neither — and the research methods have been so varied that it's tough to make generalizations. However, the research does suggest that weight gain linked to marriage is on the order of a few pounds. For instance, in a study of 9,000 men and women, women who got married during a 10-year period gained about 4 pounds more than women who were married at both the start and end of the research. In this study, men who entered into marriage during the study period did not, on average, gain more weight than men who were married all along.

Why might married folks be heavier than single people? One theory is that married couples eat more frequently and eat larger portions because they often dine together. Whereas a single person might grab a sandwich while reading a magazine, then move on to the next activity, a married couple might linger at the dinner table, heaping second helpings on their plates. Another theory is that single people may make more of an effort to keep their weight down as part of a strategy to attract a mate; once they've found a spouse, the theory goes, they have less motivation to stay slim. Perhaps people exercise less after they get married because they're busy with family obligations. Also, people getting married are less likely to smoke and more likely to quit smoking, which can lead to weight gain (see Question #57). On the bright side, married people live longer, even if they are heavier.

## Question #59: Is there any truth to the theory that people tend to lose weight after getting divorced?

*The short answer:* Men tend to lose a few pounds after the breakup of a marriage, research suggests. Among women, the trends are less clear, although it appears that divorcing women are generally likely to maintain their weight.

*Researchers don't know* why getting divorced or losing a spouse might affect men more than women, but they have some guesses. One theory is that many men, even in this post-feminist era, still don't know steaming from sautéing, so when they're back out on their own, they revert to the bachelor lifestyle. "Men, especially if their wives have cooked for them, either don't eat as much or skip meals," says Jeffery Sobal, Ph.D., an associate professor in Cornell University's division of nutritional sciences, who has studied the relationship between marital status and body weight. "Divorces are harder on men when it comes to daily habits. Women eat in very much the same way after they get divorced."

Question #60: If a dietary supplement claims to "assist with weight loss" or "reduce fat absorption," how do I know if it's true?

*The short answer:* You don't. The federal government's regulations for dietary supplement labels are generally too lax to stop manufacturers from making claims that are misleading or patently false. And although the government has recently stepped up its efforts to fight fraud, its resources are too scarce to fully enforce truth-in-advertising laws.

*A supplement manufacturer can claim,* right on the label, that a pill burns fat, builds muscle, boosts metabolism, reduces fat absorption, or "reduces the conversion of carbohydrate calories to fat" without providing any evidence to the government that the supplement actually does any of those things. This has been true ever since 1994, when Congress passed and President Clinton signed the Dietary Supplement Health and Education Act (DSHEA), a law that hardly lives up to its name. With this bill, the Food and Drug Administration's authority to regulate supplement label claims was finally weakened to the point of becoming meaningless.

Dietary supplements make up a broad category that includes vitamins, minerals, enzymes, extracts from organs or glands, and herbal and botanical agents such as ephedra and ginkgo biloba. Before the early 1990s, supplements that made certain health-related claims were held to the same standards as drugs: The FDA demanded a body of published scientific evidence showing that a supplement was both safe and effective before it could be marketed. Now the FDA demands proof of neither safety nor effectiveness, essentially leaving it up to supplement manufacturers to police themselves. Not surprisingly, the number of supplements on the market has exploded — from 4,000 when the DSHEA was passed to 29,000 ten years later.

To make matters worse, manufacturers play all sorts of shell games with their brand names and formulas, frequently changing them so that existing government investigations must start from scratch. Supplement companies often close up shop after making a killing, thereby escaping fines and avoiding irate consumers who are looking for the promised "money-back guarantee."

Soon, however, consumers may have more information to go on. The FDA recently announced it would be placing letter grades — ranging from A to D — on supplement labels, indicating the quality and strength of the scientific evidence that supports each claim. It remains to be seen whether a bad grade will shame manufacturers into dropping claims that aren't backed by solid science. The FDA has also stepped up its manufacturer inspections and seized millions of dollars' worth of mislabeled products.

Not only are many current supplement labels misleading but so are a huge proportion of the print, broadcast, and Internet ads that promote supplements. Since 1990, the Federal Trade Commission, the government agency that enforces truth-in-advertising laws, has filed about 100 cases accusing companies of false and misleading weight-loss claims for dietary supplements, over-the-counter drugs, commercial weight-loss centers, weight-loss devices, and exercise equipment. Many of these cases have led to false ads (although not the products themselves) being pulled. For instance, advertising for weight-loss pills called Exercise in a Bottle and Fat Trapper Plus were so egregiously misleading that the FTC slapped manufacturers with a $10 million fine and ordered their infomercials off the airwaves. But by that time, consumers had already forked over $100 million for pills that supposedly allowed them to eat as much as they wanted and still lose weight. And the case still isn't over; the FTC has filed several additional suits against the supplements' manufacturers for allegedly continuing to violate false advertising laws.

For every misleading ad that the FTC is able to get stopped, hundreds more sprout up, especially on the Internet. An FTC report on some 300 randomly selected weight-loss ads concluded that nearly 40 percent of the ads made at least one claim that was "almost certainly false"; another 55 percent of the ads made at least one claim that was "very likely to be false." Among the most popular tactics were misleading consumer testimonials, trumped-up scientific data, and deceptive before-and-after photos. Nearly half of the ads claimed that the users could lose weight without diet and exercise. So if you see an ad for an anti-cellulite cream that claims to work "safely and naturally without exercise," use your common sense!

## Question #61: How can I be sure that a weight-loss supplement is safe?

*The short answer:* You can't, since supplement manufacturers aren't required by law to prove their products are safe before putting them on the market.

*If enough people contact* the Food and Drug Administration with complaints about the safety of a supplement and consumer organizations lobby strongly enough, the agency may decide to investigate. But before it can require warning labels on a supplement or pull a product off the market, it must prove the supplement presents a "significant or unreasonable risk of illness or injury" — an extremely lengthy, complex, and political process that typically pits consumer advocates against industry lobbyists. The battle over ephedra (see Question #63) is a prime example of how difficult it is for the government to take even the slightest action against a product that has been linked to heart attacks, seizures, psychiatric problems, and other serious — sometimes deadly — medical conditions.

Even though the government's power has been limited in recent years, you may still be better off filing a complaint with the FDA than complaining to the manufacturer if you feel you've been harmed by a supplement. That's because, unlike drug companies, dietary supplement manufacturers aren't required to track or investigate any complaints they receive about illnesses related to the use of their products. Nor do they have to pass on any complaints to the FDA.

The fact that there are no safeguards at all for dietary supplements — some of which affect the body as significantly as many drugs — means that consumers need to be especially vigilant about which supplements they take. Of course, even the FDA's safeguards for drugs are not foolproof; many pharmaceuticals have gone through the arduous approval process only to turn out later to be harmful or, in some cases, deadly. See Question #62 for tips on doing your homework.

## Question #62: If I can't believe claims on supplement labels or in advertisements, what can I do to make sure a product I buy is safe and useful?

*The short answer:* In addition to asking yourself, "Does this sound too good to be true?" you can research supplements on various trustworthy Web sites.

*You can save yourself a lot of frustration,* not to mention money, just by maintaining a healthy skepticism about the labels and ads you read. Any suggestion that a product can help you safely lose weight without any effort on your part should be a big red flag, even if the product claims to be "an incomparable triple-action formula." Don't be lured by catch phrases like "rapid weight loss" or "jump-start your metabolism" or claims that come out of left field, such as "fat loss for men only" or "fat reduction for the apple-shaped body." Certainly don't be impressed by assertions that a product has been "protected by a United States patent." Any unique product — whether it works or not — can be patented.

Even product claims such as "published clinical studies prove success" and "resulted in significant weight loss" can be trickery. That "significant" weight loss might be as little as 2 pounds — and may be due to water loss rather than fat loss.

You can check things out for yourself by researching the supplement on Medline, an online database of peer-reviewed scientific journals. True, you may not be able to make sense of scientific verbiage like "Cr(pic)3, but not CrC13, at levels of 260 micro g Cr/kg food or less were found to lower the success rate of pupation and eclosion," but you can get a sense of whether any studies on the substance have even been published and what their general conclusions have been.

Of course, it helps to have trustworthy experts sift through the often contradictory and confusing scientific literature, which is where nonprofit consumer organizations such as the Center for Science in the Public Interest (cspinet.org) come in handy. CSPI has been a relentless advocate for more accurate nutrition labels, a safer food supply, and more nutritious food products. The organization's enlightening, reader-friendly newsletter often exposes bogus supplements as well as supermarket and restaurant foods that are shockingly unhealthful. (They're the ones who revealed that a slice of carrot cake at the Cheesecake Factory contains 1,560 calories.) The nonprofit American Council on Exercise (acefitness.org) is also a good source for honest information on supplements, as well as fitness products.

The FDA's Web site (fda.org) can update you on any governmental action that has been taken on individual supplements or on the nation's food and drug laws, and the diet and fitness pages on the FTC's site (ftc.gov/dietfit) can alert you about any pending or settled cases between the government and weight-loss product manufacturers.

Absolutely do not trust what you read on Web sites that sell supplements. The ads for pills, patches, creams, wraps, and other weight-loss products are almost uniformly misleading, if not outright false.

Question #63: Even though ephedra has been banned by the federal government, many people are still taking it. Is ephedra really unsafe?

*The short answer:* Yes. Ephedra can lead to all sorts of serious — sometimes fatal — health problems, including heart attacks, seizures, and strokes.

*In 2003,* 23-year-old Baltimore Orioles pitcher Steve Bechler collapsed of heat stroke during spring training and died the next day. Toxicology reports indicated that Bechler's death was caused, in part, by significant amounts of a supplement that contained ephedra, a stimulant he'd been taking to lose weight. Bechler's wasn't the first death linked to ephedra, which is derived from the Chinese herb ma huang, but it was the most high-profile, and it intensified the long-simmering controversy over this stimulant. In 2004, after more than a decade of lobbying by consumer health advocates and protests by the supplement industry, the Food and Drug Administration finally made the sale of ephedra illegal.

It was a government-commissioned review of ephedra research that provided some of the final nails in ephedra's coffin. An expert panel considered more than 16,000 "adverse events" reported after ephedra use and scrutinized all of the published studies on ephedra and ephedrine, ephedra's main active ingredient. Although the vast majority of complaints could not definitively be linked to use of ephedra supplements, the panel did find about 20 incidents, including heart attacks, strokes, and deaths, that they concluded could not be explained by anything other than ephedra. What's more, results from some 50 published studies suggest that ephedra users are two to three times more likely than nonusers to experience side effects such as heart palpitations, anxiety, insomnia, tremors, and stomach upset. Some of these symptoms may even show up a few weeks or months after you've gone off the supplement. Plus, users may experience withdrawal effects such as depression, exhaustion, increased appetite — even weight gain, the very thing they were trying to avoid by taking it in the first place. The risks of taking ephedra can increase with the dose, with strenuous exercise, and in conjuction with other stimulants, such as caffeine.

## Question #64: Can ephedra help me lose weight or improve my athletic performance?

*The short answer:* For all the risks ephedra poses (see Question #63), not to mention the uncomfortable side effects, the rewards are likely to be quite modest at best. Research shows that, in the short term, ephedra users lose about ½ a pound a week more than people taking placebo pills; no studies have lasted longer than six months. On the performance front, the few published studies suggest that benefits are, at best, very short-term and minimal.

*A review of 20 studies* found that over the course of about four months, people who consumed supplements containing ephedra or ephedrine and caffeine lost about 2 pounds a month more than subjects who took placebo pills. Remove the caffeine, and ephedra appears to be useless, except in high doses. Since no ephedra or ephedrine study has lasted longer than six months, long-term benefits are unknown.

Don't count on ephedra to boost your strength or cardiovascular fitness, either. Only a small number of controlled studies have been conducted, mostly on supplements containing both ephedra and caffeine and primarily on small samples of fit males, and the results were not especially impressive. In one study, for instance, ephedra boosted the number of bench press and leg press repetitions the subjects could perform, but only by a few reps and only during the first of three sets. Since virtually all of the studies on ephedra and athletic performance have tested single bouts of exercise, it is unknown whether regular use of the supplement would affect fitness over time, but given the single-bout results, it is unlikely.

The bottom line: There's no good reason to take this stuff and plenty of good reasons not to.

## Question #65: Is there any dietary supplement that can safely help me lose weight for good?

*The short answer:* No, the magic bullet simply doesn't exist.

*Given the hundreds* of weight-loss supplements hawked in health food stores and in media ads and given the boldness of their claims — "instant cellulite eraser" and "proven to emulsify fat on contact" — you might expect there to be at least a handful of products worth trying. Actually, experts say, there isn't. "In the doses advertised, none of the products have been found to be effective," says David Levitsky, Ph.D., a Cornell University nutrition professor who has studied supplements extensively. And in higher doses, he says, the supplements that might aid with short-term weight loss are potentially dangerous, increasing the risk of high blood pressure and heart problems. (Ephedra is among them; see Question #63 for details.) Not a single supplement, even any of the potentially risky ones, has been shown to have any long-term effect on weight loss.

Levitsky scrutinized 150 Web sites selling weight-loss supplements and hunted down any published scientific studies that had been conducted on the listed ingredients. Pyruvate, chromium, l-carnitine — he looked at them all. In every case, he says, either the studies did not exist or did not offer credible proof for weight-loss claims.

What about your friend who lost 10 pounds after taking a chitosan supplement and swears by it? Don't jump on the bandwagon. Some of these products, particularly those that contain herbal ingredients, cause water loss, tricking you into thinking you are getting slimmer. Others are gastrointestinal irritants; at high doses they'll make you vomit, but at low doses, they might kill your appetite by making you feel slightly ill.

In addition, there's a tremendous placebo effect with weight-loss products, especially when a supplement makes you feel different. For instance, some ingredients may make your face feel flushed or make your heart race, even if the ingredient is doing bupkis to help you shed pounds. "When you want to believe a product is working, you interpret various signals in different ways," Levitsky says. You may snack less, eat smaller portions, and make other behavior changes that will result in weight loss and then mistakenly attribute the good results to the pills you took.

If you have $50 to put toward your weight-loss efforts, don't waste it on supplements. Instead, invest the money in something that can make a real difference, such as few pairs of dumbbells, an exercise tube, a jump rope, a workout log, a subscription to *Cooking Light,* a running or cycling club membership, a pedometer, or a session with a personal trainer who can expand your repertoire of exercises.

## Question #66: How do prescription weight-loss drugs work?

*The short answer:* Most weight-loss drugs on the market are stimulants that suppress your appetite or reduce the amount of fat your body absorbs.

*There are three major drugs* currently prescribed by physicians for long-term weight loss. Each influences your ability to lose weight in a different way. The drugs also vary in their effectiveness and their side effects, as we explain in Questions #67 and 68.

The most commonly prescribed weight-loss drug is the appetite suppressant phentermine, dispensed under the brand names of Adipex and Lonamin and also as generic phentermine HCL. Phentermine works by disrupting the transmission of signals from brain chemicals known as neurotransmitters, thus tricking your brain into thinking you're not hungry.

Phentermine is the second half of the notorious drug combination fen-phen, the first half being fenfluramine. Together, the two drugs can cause serious heart-valve damage and lung problems, and fenfluramine was pulled off the market in 1997. Phentermine alone was not implicated in the health problems (though it has been linked to increased risk of stroke and heart disease), and doctors continue to prescribe it.

Sibutramine, sold under the brand name Meridia, is another commonly prescribed appetite suppressant. It controls appetite by inhibiting the uptake of the hormones serotonin, dopamine, and norepinephrine by the brain. It's similar in chemical composition to an antidepressant but affects your body and appetite in a way similar to phentermine and other stimulants. This drug seems to affect the brain's appetite-control centers by increasing feelings of fullness and satisfaction after a meal, reducing the urge to binge. (An interesting side note about the discovery of Meridia: It was originally used as an antidepressant. When researchers noticed that patients steadily lost weight while they were taking it, its manufacturers quickly repositioned it as a weight-loss drug.)

The third commonly prescribed weight-loss drug is the so-called "fat-blocker" orlistat, usually sold under the name Xenical. Xenical works in the digestive system by blocking about one-third of the fat you eat from being digested. This undigested fat is then eliminated from your body.

## Question #67: How effective are prescription weight-loss drugs?

*The short answer:* Weight-loss drugs prescribed by a doctor seem to be modestly effective. Some people who take these drugs while also following strict diet and exercise regimens drop as much as 10 percent of their body weight and keep it off for one to two years, but not all people respond to the medications. Compared with placebo-treated patients on diet and exercise alone, the drugs seem to cause, on average, an extra 5 to 15 pounds of weight loss. To maintain a lower weight, you probably have to keep taking the drugs indefinitely, and the safety of doing that is unknown.

*Cutting calories* and working out are the cornerstones of successful weight loss. Few people beyond the quacks hawking the latest fat whacker or ab melter would argue this point. Yet some people find they need extra help sticking with a healthy eating plan. This is where prescription weight-loss drugs come in. Although many doctors believe that weight-loss drugs aren't effective enough and have too many side effects to justify their use, the American Society of Bariatric Physicians and a panel of weight-loss clinic directors convened by the Institute of Medicine of the National Academies consider these drugs to have an important place in long-term weight management, at least for certain people. (See Question #69 to find out if you're a candidate for these drugs.) Drugs alone won't cause you to lose weight, but they may help control your urges so you can make better food choices.

But just how much of a difference can popping a pill with every meal make? Studies of the appetite suppressant sibutramine (Meridia) show that it has, at best, a small effect on weight loss. In studies lasting up to two years, many subjects on sibutramine were able to maintain all of their weight loss as long as they remained on the drug. However, the dropout rate for treatment with the drug is high — up to 75 percent of participants in many studies — and in order to stave off weight gain, some subjects had to increase their dosages to levels higher than currently approved by the Food and Drug Administration. Also, some of these results include only people who responded to the drug, so they don't give the complete picture.

The most commonly prescribed appetite suppressant, phentermine, has been shown to be modestly effective but use is recommended for only six months or less. Studies show that over that time, subjects on a diet plan plus phentermine lost on average 5 to 22 pounds more than subjects on a diet plan who took a placebo. However, in many studies, at the six-month mark some patients stopped losing weight and some began to regain weight even while continuing to take the drug. Results have been somewhat better in real-life settings, when the drug is prescribed in combination with diet and exercise and the patient is carefully monitored by a physician.

The fat-blocker orlistat (Xenical) has also been shown in studies to be modestly effective. Subjects on orlistat who completed trials lasting up to one year lost about 9 percent of their body weight, while subjects taking a placebo pill but following a similar weight-loss program (either a diet program or a diet-plus-exercise plan) lost 5.8 percent of their weight. Orlistat has also been found to slow the rate of regain during the second year of use. Studies show that subjects on orlistat regained 35 percent of the weight they lost, whereas subjects who lost weight through diet and exercise alone regained about 62 percent of their weight.

Unlike the stimulant diet drugs, orlistat actually has proven health benefits, such as decreased blood pressure, blood sugar, cholesterol, and triglycerides. This is in contrast to stimulants, which raise blood pressure and have not been shown to improve disease risk factors, except for slight benefits in diabetics. Orlistat does have its downsides, however. Besides its unpleasant side effects, described in Question #68, orlistat prevents absorption of fat-soluble vitamins A, E, and K, so supplements may be necessary.

So which drug is the most effective? Orlistat may be the best choice if you are concerned about lowering your heart-disease risk factors and improving your overall health. Purely in terms of weight loss, there's no clear answer, since people respond differently to different weight-loss medications. Some obese patients lose as much as 10 percent of their body weight — enough, studies suggest, to reduce risk factors for obesity-related diseases such as high blood pressure and diabetes. But others don't respond at all. Maximum weight loss usually happens within six months of starting treatment, at which point patients tend to plateau or start regaining weight. If you don't lose at least 4 pounds after four weeks on a particular drug, studies suggest, that drug is unlikely to help you. During the course of your treatment, your doctor may switch drugs or place you on a combination of drugs.

Just know that all of the drugs have side effects (see Question #68) and the likelihood of weight regain once you stop taking any of these medications is high, especially since most people tend to revert back to the behavior that caused them to carry the extra weight in the first place. Also, while you're in weight-loss drug therapy, your diet drug is only as good as your complete weight-loss program. Make sure that you are seeing a doctor who addresses your entire lifestyle rather than one who simply dispenses drugs and sends you on your way. Indeed, studies show that weight-loss drugs are far more effective when combined with a structured diet, a consistent exercise program, and behavior-modification training.

## Question #68: How safe are weight-loss drugs?

*The short answer:* In the short term, the side effects can range from dry mouth to dizzy spells to dangerously high blood pressure. Few studies have looked at safety after one year.

*Appetite suppressants* such as sibutramine and phentermine can cause symptoms ranging from dry mouth to headaches to constipation. If you take orlistat and eat a diet that's more than about 30 percent fat, you may wind up with — how shall we put this? — unpleasant stools. And of course, one of the worst side effects may be that your wallet goes on a diet right along with you: Drug therapy can cost up to $4 per day, which may or may not be covered by insurance.

It goes without saying you should never even consider taking any of these diet drugs without consulting your doctor. Although you can get a prescription and buy weight-loss drugs over the Internet with a few clicks of your mouse, this is a dangerous proposition. When taking this or any type of medication, the most important consideration should be your medical history — not your Visa number.

## Question #69: How do I know if I'm a good candidate for taking a weight-loss drug?

*The short answer:* According to the American Society of Bariatric Physicians and the National Institutes of Health, the best candidates for weight-loss drugs are people with a BMI of 30 to 39 who have tried to lose weight numerous times before and failed.

*Some physicians* also consider weight-loss drug therapy a viable option for people in the 25-to-29 BMI range who have two or more obesity-related medical conditions such as Type 2 diabetes, high blood pressure, or heart disease. Women and men with waist circumference measurements larger than 35 and 40, respectively, and who have medical problems related to their excess adipose may be considered for drug therapy as well. However, some experts oppose the use of weight-loss drugs for anyone, maintaining that the benefits are too few to warrant the risks.

## Question #70: How exactly does weight-loss surgery work?

*The short answer:* Although there are different types of weight-loss surgery procedures, all involve restricting the amount of food your stomach can hold. Some procedures also limit the number of calories your body absorbs.

*Weight-loss,* or bariatric, surgery is classified into two categories: gastric bypass and gastroplasty. To understand how these procedures work you need a brief anatomy tour. The gastrointestinal (GI) tract is essentially a 30-foot-long tube that stretches the length of your body from your mouth to your anus. Along the way, it divides up into four areas of specialized function.

From your throat, food travels down your esophagus and into your stomach, where the breakdown of food begins. You start to absorb some of the calories and nutrients as the muscles of the stomach and its digestive acids and enzymes churn food into a partially digested mush. This mush is then squeezed out of the stomach and into the first part of the small intestine, where you continue digestion and the absorption of nutrients. The 20 feet or so of remaining small intestine is where you complete digestion and absorb most of your calories and nutrients. The nondigested remnants are then dumped into the large intestine, a.k.a. the colon, where they remain until they are excreted.

Gastric-bypass procedures both limit the amount of food your stomach can hold and prevent some calories from being absorbed. These procedures involve stapling or placing a band across the upper part of the stomach to create a small stomach pouch and then rerouting a section of the small intestine to connect with the pouch. The remaining section of the small intestine, which carries bile from the liver and gallbladder as well as pancreatic enzymes, is routed back to the intestine some distance from the stomach.

The creation of the smaller stomach pouch limits the amount of food you're able to eat at any one time to just a few ounces (about the size of a shot glass), compared with the 40 ounces (about the size of a small cantaloupe) or so that a normal stomach holds. The rerouting of the small intestine allows some amount of the food you eat to bypass some portions of the digestive system that absorb calories. The percentage of calories you don't absorb depends upon the specific procedure you've undergone. The surgery is also designed to give you unpleasant symptoms or pain if you eat too much or too fast.

Gastroplasty, often called stomach stapling, refers to a group of procedures that involve placing a series of staples across the stomach. The tiny pouch fills up quickly so you feel full or nauseous after eating only a small amount of food. The pouch created in gastroplasty is essentially the same as the gastric-bypass pouch except that it's reinforced with an inflexible prosthetic ring to keep the staples from coming undone (although they *can* come undone anyway). Some newer modifications of gastroplasty, called gastric banding, create a pouch by encircling the upper stomach with a silicone band. The band can be tightened or loosened at a later date.

About 85 percent of procedures performed in the United States fall under the gastric-bypass heading. They're more popular because, as we explain in Question #71, they have a better success rate for weight loss. With gastroplasty, the staples can come undone or the bands can loosen, and the results aren't as dramatic. However, some patients still opt for gastroplasty because it's reversible, except in the case where permanent bands are installed.

Doctors warn that weight-loss surgery of any type is by no

means the easy way out. The surgery carries significant risks (see Question #73), and it doesn't let you off the hook as far as making sensible food choices. Nor does it negate the need for exercise. Once you've undergone a procedure, you have to commit to a lifetime of careful meal planning, taking specialized supplements to prevent malnutrition, and regular follow-up visits to your doctor. You can also stretch the limits of your stomach pouch, and over time, it may eventually stretch back to its original size.

## Question #71: What's the success rate of weight-loss surgery?

*The short answer:* That depends on which procedure you undergo and how committed you are to changing your eating and exercise habits.

*Given all the media attention* paid to celebrities who have slimmed to half their previous size, you might get the impression that procedures like gastric bypass are a sure-fire way to turn a fat Al Roker into a skinny Al Roker. But the reality isn't as dramatic. "Weight-loss surgery takes people who are overweight and makes them less overweight," says Louis Flancbaum, M.D., chief of bariatric surgery at St. Luke's–Roosevelt Hospital Center in New York City. "Only about 5 percent of those who have a procedure reach their ideal weight."

No national organization tracks the success of weight-loss surgery, but Flancbaum keeps statistics on the more than 8,000 patients who have undergone the procedures at his hospital. He says that success depends on which procedure you've had, how diligent you are about changing your lifestyle, and what your definition of success is.

Most gastroplasty patients lose 25 to 40 percent of their body weight within the first year and a half after surgery. Within three to five years, they typically gain back between 20 and 50 percent of their initial loss (some experts say the rate of regain is even higher). Typically this is because of an increase in calorie intake, due to the expansion of both the stomach pouch and the outlet from the stomach to the intestine.

Flancbaum thinks the weight regain is typically due to relaxed eating habits and limited food choices. Gastroplasty patients can't eat heavy or fatty meat dishes, anything with skin or seeds, or fibrous vegetables without getting violently ill; the rigid reinforcement around the stapling causes such foods to stop up the opening between the stomach and the esophagus like a clogged drain. However, foods like ice cream and candy bars easily pass through the opening. Also, because this procedure limits only food intake, not the absorption of calories, Flancbaum feels this gives gastroplasty patients a disadvantage compared with gastric-bypass patients.

The most successful gastric-bypass patients tend to lose 35 to 50 percent of their original body weight within 18 months of surgery. They, too, usually experience a weight gain within three to five years due to relaxed eating habits and adaptation within the gastrointestinal tract. Some patients may regain 10 to 15 percent of their original weight loss, while others may regain significantly more.

At least 10 percent of those who undergo any type of weight loss surgery see no results at all. Flancbaum says that failure is often due to technical reasons, such as staples coming undone. He also says that only a very small percentage of patients gain all of their weight back.

## Question #72: How do I know if I'm a good candidate for weight-loss surgery?

*The short answer:* Being overweight isn't enough. You must be diagnosed with clinically severe obesity. Typically, this is defined as having a BMI over 40 and/or being more than 100 pounds over what medical experts consider the normal weight range for your body.

*There are some exceptions* to this definition. For instance, even if you are less than 100 pounds overweight and have a BMI under 40 (but greater than 35), you may be considered a candidate if you also have serious obesity-related health complications, such as Type 2 diabetes. Most doctors who perform weight-loss surgery will reject candidates who suffer from long-term eating disorders, regardless of their weight, or who do not demonstrate a willingness to commit to lifestyle changes and lifelong follow-up visits.

### Question #73: What are the risks associated with weight-loss surgery?

*The short answer:* Most post-surgery difficulties aren't life-threatening, but this is not a surgical procedure to be taken at all lightly. One in 200 patients dies due to complications from surgery, and about 20 percent need additional surgery due to complications or failure to lose weight.

*Although gastric bypass* is booming in popularity — it seems like half the network TV shows feature an actor who has undergone this procedure — weight-loss surgery is hardly simple or risk-free. It's more serious than gallbladder surgery or appendectomy; in terms of blood loss and the reattachment of internal structures, gastric bypass is on a par with the removal of large cancers. You should have a lengthy discussion with your doctor about the risks involved.

A small percentage of patients experience complications when parts that are stapled together don't hold. For instance, the contents of the intestines can leak into the stomach, leading to erosion of internal organs or ulcer-like infections. Over time, patients are also susceptible to protein deficiencies, vitamin and mineral deficiencies, and electrolyte imbalance. These problems are especially prevalent with gastric bypass, since this procedure limits food absorption, and they can take five years or more to develop.

Question #74: What can I do about the loose skin I'm left with after losing weight?

*The short answer:* For most people, surgery is the only solution.

**When you lose 50 pounds** or more, whether on your own or through surgery, you may be left with loose hanging skin in certain areas of your body. The longer you were overweight and the older you are, the more your skin has been stretched and the less elastic it is. "By the time you hit your late forties, skin will always have trouble bouncing back after weight loss," says Al Aly, M.D., FACS, an associate professor of plastic surgery at the University of Iowa, one of the largest excess-skin-removal programs in the country.

But even young people who have gained and then lost extremely large amounts of weight — say, more than 200 pounds — will not see their skin shrink back into a nice little package again. "Think of your skin as a balloon," Aly says. "When you fill it up too far and then deflate it, it gets stretched past its normal limits, losing a lot of its original shape and elasticity."

Although the location of loose skin varies from person to person, it's especially common under the chin, on the underside of the upper arms, on the sides of the chest and midsection, and on the knees. Almost everyone who has lost a large amount of weight develops a "panniculus," an apron of skin that hangs down from the belly. Some people develop two of them, one on each side of the waist.

Exercise is important for toning your body after weight loss, but it's not going to tone up your skin. The only remedy for overstretched skin appears to be surgery. In the case of the middle-body apron, this means a tummy tuck or, if skin hangs around the entire middle, a belt lipectomy. During a belt lipectomy, the surgeon cuts away the draping or loose skin and tightens up the underlying muscles in an effort to prevent hernias and minimize roundness. "You don't get good results when you just remove the skin," Aly says. "You also need to tighten up the patient's 'inner balloon of musculature' to get good results."

Not everyone is a good candidate for this type of surgery. Surgeons generally won't operate on anyone who smokes, who hasn't been at a stable weight for at least six months, or who has a heart condition, diabetes, lung disease, or a diagnosed psychological disorder. Recovery from these operations typically takes 4 to 6 weeks, although it's important for patients to get up and moving as soon as possible, ideally within hours of surgery, to prevent circulation problems and blood clotting. Although considered cosmetic surgery, these operations are nevertheless major surgery and carry a risk of complications, including fatal clots.

## Question #75: What happens if I regain all the weight back after I've had excess skin removed?

*The short answer:* Your skin stretches again.

*If you were to regain hundreds of pounds* after having a tummy tuck, belt lipectomy, or other skin removal procedure (see Question #74), you would be in no danger of bursting out of your remaining skin. "Skin has a great elastic ability," says University of Iowa plastic surgeon Al Aly. "It would simply expand to accommodate the extra weight." However, Aly notes, it is extremely rare for people to regain substantial amounts of weight after going through the trouble of having excess skin removed.

## Question #76: How exactly does liposuction work, and is it safe?

*The short answer:* Liposuction involves sucking out body fat with a hollow metal rod, called a cannula, that's attached to a vacuum. When performed by a qualified, experienced surgeon, the procedure is quite safe.

*The horror stories* reported during the early days of liposuction are essentially a thing of the past. These days you don't hear about patients left with deep ridges on their skin as if a rake had been dragged across their thighs or, far worse, patients dying after having enormous amounts of fat vacuumed from their bodies. Improved techniques and state government regulations limiting the amount of fat that can be removed during surgery have made liposuction a low-risk procedure, at least when it's performed by an experienced board-certified plastic surgeon.

Just be aware that any doctor can perform liposuction, and some who do it lack adequate training. And even under the best of circumstances, liposuction, like any surgical procedure, has its risks. The more fat removed, the greater the risk. Although very rare, these risks include excess bleeding, infection, and excessive fluid loss leading to shock. Potential side effects include bruising, permanent changes in skin color, and permanently ripply skin. Also, when it's performed by a doctor who is less than a pro, liposuction can result in an asymmetrical appearance, a good reason to thoroughly check out your physician before you submit to a procedure.

Probably the greatest advance in liposuction is the tumescent technique. The doctor injects the patient's targeted area with a saline solution mixed with adrenaline and a local anesthetic. This causes the fat cells to swell — "tumesce" — and the blood vessels to constrict. As a result, "the fat almost pours out," as one surgeon told us, and patients bleed very little during surgery. Afterward, they experience less bruising and swelling than when liposuction is performed without the tumescent solution.

For larger volumes of fat or fat that is particularly dense and fibrous, many doctors insert an ultrasound probe underneath the skin to liquefy the fat before it is suctioned.

## Question #77: Is liposuction a good idea if I don't have that much weight to lose?

*The short answer:* Liposuction isn't designed for weight loss. If you turn to surgery because it seems a lot easier than exercising and skipping dessert, you'll probably gain those bulges right back. The best candidates are people who already work out and eat sensibly but have stubborn pockets of fat that still won't budge.

*For some people,* all the exercise and nutritional improvements won't eliminate those saddlebags or that plump neck that runs in the family. These are the patients whom liposuction doctors prefer because they have a good chance of maintaining their post-lipo physique. Patients who use liposuction as a weight-loss shortcut tend to be repeat customers because they regain the fat. If you have liposuction repeatedly, you're likely to end up with scar tissue that makes each subsequent procedure more difficult for the doctor to perform.

Liposuction isn't as simple as submitting to an outpatient procedure and then slipping into a smaller bathing suit. If you do have lipo, you won't be able to exercise for two to four weeks. You also may not be able to shower, since you'll have to wear a compression stocking around the area that was treated. You'll also be sore and bruised for those first few weeks. Make sure you get right back on that treadmill as soon as you're cleared by your doctor. Otherwise, as we explain in Question #78, you could potentially be back to square one.

## Question #78: What are the chances of regaining weight after liposuction?

*The short answer:* There are no solid published studies that track long-term success of liposuction patients after surgery.

*As any responsible plastic surgeon* will tell you, having excess fat sucked out of your body is not an unconditional ticket to a life of gluttony and sloth. True, the fat cells that have been removed can't grow back, but the billions of fat cells still in your body still have the capacity to expand. (And actually, in animal studies, new fat cells have formed to replace ones that are removed surgically, although they usually sprout up elsewhere in the body.) If you don't watch your eating and exercise habits after liposuction, you can still regain weight.

Plastic surgeons report, anecdotally, that most of their patients are highly motivated to keep their figures after surgery, so they eat nutritiously and work out regularly. However, since little research has been published on success rates, nobody knows for sure how liposuction patients fare years down the line. Also, published reports may include only a doctor's most successful cases, as patients who have regained weight may not be eager to stay in touch.

## Question #79: If I do gain weight after liposuction, where will the fat go?

*The short answer:* Doctors don't know where weight gain after liposuction is most likely to pop up; the question has barely been addressed in research. However, many surgeons say, patients who gain weight after surgery will probably accumulate a greater portion of fat in non-suctioned regions of the body.

*The location of regained fat* isn't just a question of aesthetics; it could potentially impact a patient's health. For instance, if a patient who has fat sucked from her hips regains fat deep in the abdomen, it's possible that such a redistribution could negatively impact her cholesterol levels, insulin sensitivity (defined in Question #211), and other cardiovascular disease risk factors. "It could be a potential problem in a select number of patients, but we don't have enough information about it, and it probably would not affect patients across the board," says Peter Rubin, M.D., an assistant professor of plastic surgery at the University of Pittsburgh Medical Center. Rubin is currently conducting a study using CT scanning to track the amount and location of fat in patients three months and eight months after liposuction. Rubin's research may shed more light on the issue, since he is monitoring the effect of liposuction on blood fat levels, insulin sensitivity, metabolism, and hormone levels.

Interestingly, anecdotal reports and one published study suggest that some women, primarily those who have had large volumes of fat removed from the abdominal area and then regain weight, experience breast enlargement in the months following liposuction. However, it is not known whether the growth represents fat or lean breast tissue, what causes it, or how common this phenomenon may be.

If liposuction patients keep off the fat, might their cardiovascular risk profile improve? One study of 14 moderately overweight liposuction patients found decreases in blood pressure and fasting insulin levels (a measure of diabetes risk) four months after surgery. However, another study found that liposuction did not lower diabetes or heart disease risk in obese women who lost up to 23 pounds of belly fat.

It's likely that liposuction affects patients in different ways, since human fat patterns vary so much and fat cells in different areas of the body behave very differently. Considering how popular liposuction has become — more than 150,000 procedures are performed each year — physicians know relatively little about the effects of the surgery in the long run.

## Question #80: I heard that obesity can be caused by a virus. Could this possibly be true?

*The short answer:* As farfetched as it sounds, there is mounting evidence that in some cases, obesity can be caught like the common cold. At this point the idea is theoretical in humans. However, scientists have isolated at least seven viruses that definitively cause obesity in birds, dogs, and monkeys, and some of those viruses are also known to infect humans.

*Back in the 1970s,* scientists in India began studying a viral disease that was killing chickens by the thousands. Infected birds didn't waste away as they got sicker; instead they packed on pounds — up to 50 percent more fat tissue than uninfected birds. Oddly, the sick chickens also tested low for levels of cholesterol and triglycerides (fat in the bloodstream). Normally, obesity is associated with high levels of cholesterol and triglycerides. Even stranger, the infected birds did not seem to eat more as they gained weight.

The researchers isolated the cause of the birds' sickness as Adenovirus-36, or Ad-36, a highly infectious microbe that causes colds, diarrhea, and pinkeye in humans. Dozens of human and animal adenoviruses are known to exist. Researchers wondered: Could Ad-36 as well as other, similar viruses contribute to the obesity epidemic in humans?

"We're 100 percent certain that viral infections cause obesity in animals but can only infer that it causes obesity in people, since we can't ethically test the theory on human subjects," says Nikhil Dhurandhar, Ph.D., obesity research chair in the department of nutrition and food sciences at Wayne State University in Detroit, Michigan.

Still, the case for an obesity-causing human virus is bolstered by nearly 100 studies done over the last 35 years or so and has recently piqued the interest of mainstream obesity researchers. For example, a group of four studies done at the University of Wisconsin at Madison have caught the attention — and respect — of the scientific community. One such investigation tested people for the existence of Ad-36 antibodies in their blood. An antibody is a chemical produced by the body to fight a particular condition; its presence is a sort of biological fingerprint that proves a person was infected with Ad-36 at some point. More than 30 percent of the obese subjects tested positive for Ad-36 antibodies, compared with only 5 percent of normal-weight individuals.

When the researchers factored out 29 other possible causes of weight gain, such as genetics, family history, and lifestyle, the two groups did not differ in any other respects. The Ad-36-positive subjects were among the most obese in the study, yet paradoxically had low cholesterol and triglyceride levels — just like the chickens in India. German researchers who studied nearly 100 pairs of twins found that when one twin tested positive for Ad-36 antibodies, that twin always had a higher percentage of body fat than the non-infected twin.

Experts are not completely surprised by the Wisconsin researcher's results. In the past few years, scientists have found that many chronic health conditions once thought to have other causes are linked to biological infections. For instance, scientists long thought that most ulcers were caused by high stress and poor diet, not a bacterial infection; but now the ulcer bug, *Helicobacter pylori,* is accepted as reality and ulcers are most commonly treated with antibiotics.

So how could a virus cause obesity? Scientists speculate that Ad-36 increases the number and size of adipocytes (fat cells) by stimulating more immature fat cells to bloom more quickly into full-fledged fat cells. Evidence suggests that animals infected with Ad-36 may wind up with 3 times more adipocytes than uninfected animals. Adenoviruses may decrease metabolism as well.

But before you start edging away from that overweight individual in the elevator when he sneezes, a lot more investigation needs to be done. If Ad-36 is shown to cause excessive weight gain in humans, it's not clear how it spreads or how contagious it may be, especially once the person has already reached corpulence. It's also unclear how many other human viruses may have similar effects. The number of people tested is still too small to determine how many people are infected and what percentage of those who are develop obesity as a symptom.

Still, many experts believe that skyrocketing worldwide obesity rates can't be totally explained by super-sized portions and a couch-potato lifestyle, and that viruses may be a contributing factor. The Wayne State research team, led by Dhurandhar, has received a National Institutes of Health grant to further investigate the concept of "infectobesity." Also, several other research teams around the world are studying this issue.

Even if viruses are responsible for some cases of obesity, Dhurandhar points out that the cure remains the same: Eat less, move more.

## Question #81: What is leptin, and what does it have to do with weight loss?

*The short answer:* Leptin, a hormone released by your fat cells, is among the body's chemicals responsible for controlling appetite, storing fat, and regulating your body's ability to burn fat. Scientists have found that many overweight and obese people have a surplus of leptin in the bloodstream, suggesting that some sort of leptin resistance or malfunction may contribute to weight gain.

*Leptin* (from the Greek word *leptos*, meaning "thin") was discovered in the late 1990s by researchers at Rockefeller University in New York City. Investigators found that some mice predisposed to super-obesity had a genetic defect preventing leptin production. When the mice were injected with leptin, they experienced dramatic weight loss virtually overnight. Remarkably, they lost only body fat, leaving lean tissue untouched.

The leptin curbed their appetites and kick-started their sluggish metabolisms, causing researchers to wonder: Could they be on the path to an effective new weight-loss treatment for humans?

Alas, as with many animal experiments, the results didn't translate to humans. Turns out, most overweight people have an excess, rather than an absence, of leptin in their bloodstreams. At first scientists were puzzled. They expected high levels of leptin to correspond to better appetite control, faster fat burning, and speedier metabolism. But upon further research they discovered that, while obese people do have high leptin levels, their bodies seem unable to process it. No matter how much of the stuff the body pumps out, it's not enough to suppress appetite or accelerate metabolism.

So where does leptin research fit into the fight against obesity? Many medical experts believe the existence of leptin shows that, for some people, the drive to devour junk food may have a biological basis — that it's not simply lack of willpower that makes some of us reach for fries, doughnuts, and other high-fat, high-calorie foods.

Current leptin research is focused on how weight loss affects leptin levels and leptin resistance. Preliminary findings show that when people lose weight, their leptin levels return to normal and the body's ability to process leptin is restored. Exercise without weight loss also seems to enhance leptin balance, although at this point that's just a theory. In any case, researchers hope the studies will offer a promising new direction for the development of obesity and weight-loss drugs. In the meantime, resist the urge to buy leptin supplements over the Web. They're as much of a scam as any slimming patch or fat burner being sold.

### Question #82: How do sumo wrestlers get so fat, and how unhealthy are they?

*The short answer:* Sumo wrestlers get fat the same way other people do — by eating enormous portions of high-calorie fare. The life expectancy of a sumo wrestler is less than 60 years, far lower than the Japanese male average of 80 years. Many are plagued by weight-related problems such as difficulty walking, osteoarthritis, and high blood pressure. However, in spite of their belt-popping girth, sumo wrestlers are healthier than you might expect.

*Top sumo wrestlers* are among some of the weightiest individuals on earth. On average they tip the scales at 400 pounds — some weigh in at more than 600 pounds — with an average body mass index of 36.5 and body-fat percentage of 30.

By virtually every standard measure, these large men in diapers are considered obese. But they probably aren't as unhealthy as your typical burger-and-fries-addicted couch potato. Studies show elite sumo wrestlers tend to have normal cholesterol, glucose, and triglyceride levels. As a group, they don't suffer inordinately from heart disease, they rarely develop Type 2 diabetes, and they have relatively modest amounts of fat deep within the abdomen, the type of fat linked to heart disease and other health problems.

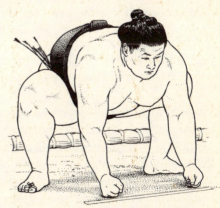

*Sumo wrestlers aren't as unhealthy as you might think.*

Medical experts speculate that sumo wrestlers enjoy comparatively good health because they exercise. A lot. Although you don't see too many sumo wrestlers jogging in the park, their training regimen calls for grueling 4- or 5-hour workouts six or seven days a week. The problems set in when these wrestlers retire; they continue eating the same way they did when they competed and begin to develop lifestyle-related diseases.

Lately there has been growing concern that sumo competitors have grown too fat. In 1953, the average sumo wrestler stood 5-foot-11 and weighed 317 pounds. Today, the average wrestler is just 3 inches taller but 95 pounds heavier, probably due to eating too much junk food and too much food, period. A few years back, the Japanese Sumo Association issued a stern warning to wrestlers who tested over 38 percent body fat, advising them to lose weight or risk being suspended from competition.

Don't expect a sportwide slim-down anytime soon. There are no weight classes in sumo wresting — a 200-pounder must compete against a 400-pounder, so sumo wrestlers have an incentive to get as big as possible by any means possible. However, the super-sized wrestlers of today aren't nearly as agile or quick on their feet as the relatively trimmer competitors of yesteryear.

## Question #83: How can I tell if my dog is overweight?

*The short answer:* When you can't see or feel his ribs or when you look at him from above and he has no waist, you're the owner of a pooch that could lose a few pounds.

*Considering that the average housedog* is basically a glorified throw rug with a pulse, it's not surprising that more than 50 percent of the 60 million dogs in America are considered overweight; 25 percent of them are considered obese. Why your little Snuffle Pumpkin is overweight should come as no surprise: too much food and too much time spent curled up on the couch.

He's susceptible to many of the same obesity-related diseases as humans are, such as diabetes and heart disease. Compared with their slimmer pack-mates, fat dogs are also more prone to injury and complications in surgery and experience more stress on their heart, lungs, liver, kidneys, and joints. A study done at the University of Pennsylvania found that overfed Labradors had their life spans shortened by 1.8 years and developed chronic conditions such as osteoarthritis at a younger age than Labs of normal weight. While this study did not factor in other doggy lifestyle factors such as amount of exercise, it does suggest that a fat pooch is an unhealthy pooch.

Once a dog weighs 15 percent more than his ideal weight, he's considered clinically obese. Veterinarians use a 9-point rating system to evaluate a dog's weight, with a score of 1 given to a dog that is extremely thin and a score of 9 given to a dog that's a real porker. Ideally, your dog should fall right in the middle, with a score of 5.

To determine your dog's body score, start by palpating his ribs. There should be a slight amount of fat over them, but you should be able to feel each rib distinctly. If you have to poke and prod through rolls of pudge, it's time to seriously consider cutting back on the Puppy Chow. Other "tell-tail" signs that your dog could use fewer kibbles and a few more walks: a great deal of excess fat covering his hipbones, spine, and shoulders and rolls of fat under his neck and limbs and at the base of his tail.

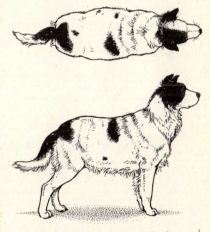

If you think your dog is overweight, consult your veterinarian to rule out any underlying medical problems before starting the animal on a weight-reduction program. Don't just cut off his food supply and put him through nightly 10-mile training runs. Dogs, like humans, need to

*Put your dog on a diet and exercise program if you can't see his ribs and his body has no curves.*

ease into healthy eating and exercise habits. Limit his weight loss to no more than 4 percent per week. Your veterinarian can help you formulate an appropriate weight-loss plan.

Some dog breeds seem to have a genetic tendency toward overly thick waistlines. These include Labrador retrievers, beagles, basset hounds, dachshunds, cocker spaniels, and Shetland sheepdogs. If your four-legged friend is one of these breeds, take extra care to make sure he gets enough exercise to work off his daily ration.

# Nutrition: Diets, Food Labels, and Eating for Exercise

B arely a week goes by when there's not a diet book on the *New York Times* bestseller list. *Atkins for Life; Sugar Busters!; The South Beach Diet; Suzanne Somers' Eat, Cheat, and Melt the Fat Away* — we seem to have quite an appetite for books about how to curb our appetites. But how much of what these diet gurus say is true?

We're not going to analyze every flavor-of-the-month eating plan in this section, but we will give you the knowledge to separate sound nutritional advice from the pseudoscience presented in many of the best-selling diet books. Although diet gurus tend to promote strict rules for eating, nutritional science has a long way to go before answering the most controversial questions, and clearly there is no single best eating plan for everyone.

In this section, we tell you what the research says thus far about low-carb diets and about whether eating high-fat foods makes you fat. We also look at what studies prove, or don't prove, about timing your eating: Will eating at night make you fat? Is it better to eat three square meals day or six smaller ones? In addition, we explain whether it helps for weight loss to eat more fiber, drink lots of water, use artificial sweeteners, and follow the glycemic index.

Of course, what you eat and when you eat affect more than your weight; your food choices also affect how energetic you feel and how well you perform when you exercise. Do you need extra protein if you lift weights? Is it okay to eat right before a workout? These and other sports nutrition questions are answered here.

## Question #84: How many calories should I eat each day?

*The short answer:* The number depends primarily on your basal metabolic rate and how active you are — and, of course, on your goals. To lose weight, you need to eat fewer calories than it takes to maintain your current weight.

*To **determine the number*** of calories necessary to maintain your weight, first estimate your basal metabolic rate (BMR), the amount of energy your body needs simply to stay alive — to keep your heart beating, your lungs expanding, your liver functioning. Your BMR accounts for 60 to 70 percent of your daily caloric burn and depends on several factors, including your height, weight, gender, age, and muscle mass. Women tend to have lower BMRs because they're smaller and typically carry a greater percentage of body fat. Older people also tend to have lower BMRs, in part because of muscle loss that comes with aging.

The easiest way to determine your BMR is to use a formula. The most common is the Harris-Benedict, named after the two scientists who created it.

**Men:** 66 + (6.3 x body weight in lbs.) + (12.9 x height in inches) – (6.8 x age in years)

**Women:** 655 + (4.3 x weight in lbs.) + (4.7 x height in inches) – (4.7 x age in years)

So if you're a 35-year-old woman who is 5-foot-5 and weighs 145 pounds, your BMR would be 1,420. (If you're math phobic, you can do a simpler calculation using the Math-Hater's Shortcut on pages 114–115. Or, plug your height, weight, and age into an on-line BMR calculator. Just know that different Web sites use different formulas, so results may vary.)

Of course, a formula can give you only an estimate. Some gyms and hospitals use machines that can more precisely estimate the number of your basic calorie needs. These machines actually measure your RMR — resting metabolic rate — a measure that's slightly higher than your BMR. Your BMR is the number of calories you need to survive; your RMR is that plus the extra calories you need when you are awake but basically inactive. For the purposes of estimating your daily calorie needs, it doesn't really matter whether you're using BMR or RMR.

You may be offered a free RMR test upon joining a club or be charged up to $100. The BodyGem, for example, requires you to breathe through your mouth into a tube for 10 minutes. The machine then analyzes the composition of the gases in your breath to give a pretty accurate estimate of your RMR, provided you haven't exercised or eaten recently. (This is different from the contraptions used in research settings, which have so many wires and dials that they look like something out of a Frankenstein movie.)

Once you have estimated the RMR or BMR portion of your daily calorie requirement, add in the calories needed for physical activity. We're not just talking about the amount of time you spend on the treadmill or the tennis court. Physical activity includes everything from walking between the phone and the fax machine to brushing your teeth to sorting out newspapers for the recycling bin. The more of these "lifestyle activity" calories you burn, the larger your calorie requirement.

To estimate how many calories you need to fuel your daily activities, multiply your BMR by the percentage that matches your activity level:

- **Sedentary** (mainly sitting all day) — 20 percent
- **Light activity** (such as walking to and from the bus stop, cooking dinner) — 30 percent
- **Moderate activity** (very little sitting, heavy housework, and gardening) — 40 percent
- **Very active** (construction work, intense or prolonged exercise) — 50 percent

So, to continue our example: If you're a 35-year-old woman with a BMR of 1,420 and your activity level is light, multiply 1,420 by .3. The result is 426. Now add the additional 426 calories you need to sustain your activity to your BMR. Your daily caloric needs are up to 1,846.

However, your actual caloric needs are slightly higher due to the "thermic effect of food," the amount of energy your body uses to digest food, breaking it down to its basic elements in order to be used by the body. For digestion processes, your body uses up 5 to 10 percent of the total calories you eat.

Keep in mind that combining your BMR, physical activity level, and calories needed for digestion give you an estimate of the calories needed to *maintain* your weight. To *lose* weight, you need to create a calorie deficit, ideally by both eating less and moving more.

In general, you shouldn't cut calories too drastically or go overboard on exercise. Otherwise, you'll lose too much muscle — plus, you're likely to fall off the wagon quickly and gain the weight right back. Instead, aim for calorie cuts and an activity boost that you can comfortably sustain. For instance, if you simply cut 125 calories a day (one large pat of butter or two small cookies) while burning an extra 125 calories through exercise (walking about 1 mile), you'll cut 1,750 calories a week — enough to lose about ½ pound. That may not sound like much, but the more slowly you lose weight, the more likely you are to keep it off. Most nutritionists recommend aiming to lose no more than ½ pound to 1 pound a week. To lose 1 pound, cut 250 calories from your diet and bump your activity level by 250 calories.

## The Math-Hater's Shortcut to Estimating Your Daily Calorie Needs

If you fear the buttons on your calculator, here's a simple way to estimate your caloric daily needs. It's not quite as precise as the Harris-Benedict formula described on page 112, but it will give you a rough estimate of the number of calories you need to eat to maintain your weight.

- **Very Light Exercise** (example: You walk less than 15 minutes per day): Multiply your weight in pounds by 13.

- **Light Exercise** (example: You walk 15 to 30 minutes five times per week): Multiply your weight in pounds by 14.

- **Moderate Exercise** (example: You walk for exercise or accumulate at least 30 minutes of low- to moderate-intensity walking during your day four or five times per week): Multiply your weight in pounds by 15.25.

- **Moderate-Heavy Exercise** (example: You get at least 45 minutes of brisk activity, at 70 percent of your maximum intensity or above, three to five times per week): Multiply your weight in pounds by 16.5.

- **Heavy Exercise** (example: You work out at a moderate to high intensity more than five times a week, 45 minutes per session): Multiply your weight in pounds by 18.

### Question #85: For weight loss, is it better to eat six small meals a day than three large ones?

*The short answer:* If the total number of calories you consume is the same, the number of meals you eat doesn't really matter. Some people can more easily control calories by eating several small meals, whereas others fare better on three squares a day.

*In theory,* eating six smaller meals is the way to go. Eating more often keeps your blood sugar on an even keel, preventing you from becoming weak and tired. More frequent eating may also keep you from becoming ravenously hungry and raiding the cookie jar. What's more, several studies have observed that people who eat more frequently, a.k.a. "nibblers," weigh less than people who eat less often, a.k.a. "gorgers." One possible reason is that the body may burn slightly more calories digesting and processing several small meals than three larger ones.

But the issue isn't so clear-cut. A *British Journal of Nutrition* article that reviewed research on meal frequency and weight concluded that, taken as a whole, the evidence is "at best very weak" that nibblers weigh less than gorgers. Equally iffy, they concluded, is the notion that the body burns more calories digesting several small meals than fewer large ones; the studies that used the most sophisticated methods found no difference in calorie expenditure between nibbling and gorging.

While nobody disputes that frequent eating keeps blood-sugar levels stable, this may not necessarily translate into better calorie control. Some people, researchers say, may actually eat more food over the course of a day given the opportunity to eat more often. And many people find it unsatisfying or inconvenient to limit their meals to, say, 330 calories (a typical 2,000-calorie-per-day diet roughly divided by six meals). This limit is probably easiest met at breakfast. For 330 calories, you can eat 2 eggs, a slice of toast, and 6 ounces of orange juice, or ¾ cup Kellogg's Raisin Bran with 1 cup of skim milk and a banana. But lunch or dinner can be tougher; 330 calories gets you a skinless chicken breast and a side of black beans. For some people this may be unsatisfying, even with a 330-calorie mini-meal a couple of hours later. (Or you could blow the whole 330 calories on a medium order of fries at McDonald's.)

You may find that three moderately sized meals plus an afternoon snack works best. The bottom line: Experiment with different meal patterns and see what works for you.

## Question #86: Is it true that any calories you eat after 6 P.M. turn to fat?

*The short answer:* No, this is an urban legend — no more true than the notion that alligators are roaming the sewers of New York City. However, late-night eating can sabotage your weight-loss program for other reasons.

*If you eat more calories* than your body burns in a day — no matter what time you eat them — the excess calories will be stored as fat. If you eat fewer calories than your body burns — even if some of those calories are consumed during *The Tonight Show* — you will lose weight. There is no intrinsic connection between calories and the clock.

But this doesn't mean nighttime eating can't sabotage your weight-loss plan. If you have a tendency to skip meals or eat lightly throughout the day, you may be more likely to stage a midnight refrigerator raid. Also, many people tend to unwind at night in front of the TV. When your eyes are glued to the tube, you're more prone to mindless munching. As you flip channels you may not even realize you're inhaling an entire bag of M&M's and a quart of soda.

## Question #87: How do scientists measure the calories contained in a certain food?

*The short answer:* They measure the amount of heat contained within its chemical bonds.

*It's a classic Biology 101 experiment:* You hold a peanut in a bent paper clip under a test tube that contains ten grams of water, then you light a match and set the peanut on fire. The peanut burns and burns and burns, then burns some more. The water in the test tube starts to boil. When the peanut has finally vanished, there are only 8 grams of water left. You now know enough, if armed with the correct formulas, to determine that the peanut contained about 18 calories.

To a scientist, a calorie is the amount of heat needed to raise the temperature of 1 gram of water by 1 degree Celsius. (More about this in Question #29.) The chemical energy contained within the nut provides fuel to heat the water. Based on the amount of time the peanut burns and how much water it brings to a boil, you can calculate how many calories are contained within the peanut — or any other food, for that matter.

Basically, that's how the science of food calorimetry works, except that instead of a paper clip and a match, labs are equipped with special heating chambers called bomb calorimeters. First a food sample is dried and ground into a fine powder, then it's placed into the bomb calorimeter, which itself is submerged in a water bath. The bomb is pumped full of pure oxygen and the food is ignited, resulting in a quick, violent release of energy — just like a bomb. The temperature increase of the water and metal of the calorimeter reveals the food's "heat of combustion." To determine the food's caloric value, scientists then factor out things like which portion of the food is indigestible.

## Question #88: What should I look for on a food label?

*The short answer:* That depends on your nutrition goals and the type of food you're looking at, but in general focus on the serving size, calories, trans and saturated fat grams, and fiber grams.

*Nutrition Facts labels* are required by the government on all packaged foods, and they're essential reading if you're trying to clean up your diet. Labels serve as a crucial counterbalance to the marketing hype and sneaky advertising tactics commonly used in food packaging.

If you're watching your weight, the first number to focus on is . . . no, not the calories but the serving size. A 75-calorie serving of chocolate chip cookies might sound like a caloric bargain, but it's hardly a good deal if a serving consists of a single miniature cookie. Keep in mind that serving sizes listed on food packages generally are much smaller than what the average person actually eats. When was the last time you measured out ½ cup of ice cream or sliced a roll in half?

The number of total fat grams listed on a food label isn't especially useful, for reasons we discuss in Question #92. However, pay attention to the amount of saturated and trans fat in a product. As we explain in Question #93, the less of these two fats the better; none is best.

The Nutrition Facts fiber information is particularly useful when you're comparing bread and cereal products. Often the packaging will suggest the product is high in fiber — you'll see pictures of wheat fields waving in the wind and names like "12 Grain Bread" or "Organic Brown Rice Crisps" — and yet a serving may contain the same amount of fiber, practically zilch, as Wonder Bread or Frosted Flakes.

Food labels also reveal the truth about the ingredients in a product, as well as the vitamin and mineral content. For example, you might think that Kern's All Nectar Strawberry Banana would be "all nectar," or at least substantially so. In reality, the product contains just 22 percent juice. Sunny Delight's Real Fruit Beverage drink contains just 5 percent juice.

The part of the food label that seems to trip people up is the term "%DV," short for Percent Daily Value. Daily Values are set by the government and reflect current nutrition recommendations for a 2,000-calorie diet. You can use the %DV to see how the amount of a nutrient in a particular food fits into an "average" diet. For instance, you can see that a bottled peach-mango smoothie may contain 35 percent of the Daily Value of vitamin C, compared with 150 percent of the Daily Value for 8 ounces of plain old orange juice. You can also see that Rice-A-Roni's Chicken & Broccoli dish contains virtually no broccoli and just 2 percent of the Daily Value of vitamin C; ½ cup chopped fresh broccoli contains 98 percent of the DV.

## Question #89: How can I find out how many calories are in foods that aren't labeled?

*The short answer:* Go to the U.S. Department of Agriculture's nutrient database, or buy any of the books on the market that list the nutrient values for thousands of foods and beverages.

*Whether you're trying to control* your weight or just eat more nutritiously, it's crucial to read the Nutrition Facts labels on food packages. At a glance you can see how many calories are in Mr. Goodbar (290 — yikes!) or how much fiber is in Kellogg's Raisin Bran (a nutritious 5 grams). But what do you do about foods that don't come with labels, like a tangerine or a bowl of spaghetti or the beef ribs at your favorite steak joint?

Not that you need to know the calorie count for every morsel of food you consume — that would take the fun out of eating — but with more information, you're likely to make better choices. One excellent resource is the USDA's National Nutrient Database for Standard Reference: nal.usda.gov/fnic/foodcomp/search. The database is more complete than many books on the subject and it's updated on a regular basis. Enter any food item, such as "beef ribs," and you may get dozens of options, from "trimmed to ¼-inch fat prime, cooked, broiled" to "trimmed to ⅛-inch fat choice, cooked, roasted." When you make your selection you not only see the number of calories, saturated fat grams, protein grams, and carb grams, you also see the various vitamin and mineral estimates.

Obviously, when you eat at a restaurant, you don't know how many grams of fat your fillet of sole is swimming in or exactly what ingredients are jumbled into your jambalaya, but gathering some general nutritional estimates from a database or book can turn you into a much more informed eater.

## Question #90: Can I trust the labels on supermarket foods or the calorie counts listed on chain-restaurant Web sites?

*The short answer:* The information coming from national brands is usually, although not always, pretty accurate. However, in spot checks, many food labels from regional brands have been found to vastly underestimate the number of calories and the amount of fat and sugar contained in the product.

*Does your favorite energy bar* actually contain the 220 calories it claims to on the label? Do those extra-lean burgers you always buy really contain just 2 grams of saturated fat per patty? Those aren't questions we normally ask. Most of us assume that Nutrition Facts labels — required by law on all processed, packaged food products and relied on by millions to make healthy food choices — reflect reality.

Turns out, many of the labels may not. In a test conducted by the Florida Department of Agriculture and Consumer Services laboratory, 75 percent of diet products tested, most of them regional brands, were shown to have erroneous information on their labels. More than 10 percent of all bakery products and candies tested were mislabeled, as were 25 percent of dressings and condiments. Some of the labels were off-the-charts misleading, like a vanilla éclair that claimed to have 2 grams of fat but actually contained 17 grams. An entire line of "sugar-free" baked goods — more than 20 products — from a regional company was found to contain sugar, as many as 16 grams per serving. Caught red-handed, one company employee admitted that sugar was added to give the chocolate products more flavor and enable the cookie dough to brown better.

Tests commissioned by the Center for Science in the Public Interest, a nonprofit consumer organization, found that Laura's Lean steaks contained, on average, more than twice as much fat and saturated fat and 40 percent more calories than the company stated. Laura's strip steaks were certified to use the American Heart Association's "heart-check" logo on their labels, yet all but one of the 14 strip steaks tested failed to meet the AHA's guidelines, which require a serving of meat to contain less than 5 grams of total fat and less than 2 grams of saturated fat. The steaks were later, um, stripped of their certification.

Although it's typically regional brands that are guilty of deception, even national corporations have on occasion been caught duping the public. Not long ago, CSPI busted McDonald's for low-balling numbers for its vanilla reduced-fat ice cream. In this case, the inaccuracy was related to serving sizes. The McDonald's Web site offered nutrition information for only a 90-gram ice cream cone, purported to have 150 calories and 3 grams of saturated fat. But the smallest cone that CSPI researchers found in the Washington, D.C., area exceeded McDonald's official size by 49 percent and contained an average of 225 calories and 4.5 grams of saturated fat.

Most state governments don't do food-product testing, the federal government rarely makes random checks, and organizations like CSPI can only do so much. So what's a consumer to do? Your best bet is to assume a modest overestimation of calories and fat grams and make your choices accordingly. Keep in mind that labels that "pass" the accuracy test may not be entirely on target. Federal law allows most products a 20 percent variance from the label; in other words, a bagel that claims to contain 200 calories legally can contain 240 calories. In addition, the government allows for a 10 percent margin of error in testing, so some labels may be as much as 30 percent off without being considered misleading. Not surprisingly, manufacturers rarely seem to err on the side of *over*estimating calories and fat.

## Question #91: Are portion sizes larger than they used to be?

*The short answer:* Big time! Cookies, muffins, candy bars, steaks, sodas, and dozens of other foods started ballooning in the 1970s, dramatically inflated in the 1980s, and have continued to expand, to the point where some food products are now five times their original size. Not surprisingly, our nation of super-sized fries has become a nation of super-sized thighs.

*Brick-sized candy bars* and cookies the diameter of a CD may seem the norm, but food portions weren't always so massive. Back in the 1950s, McDonald's offered only one size of French fries. That size, containing 210 calories, is now the smallest of three sizes offered; the largest contains 520 calories. (McDonald's recently nixed its 610-calorie super-sized fries.) The 7-Eleven Double Gulp, a 64-ounce soda (nearly 800 calories) is 10 times the size of a Coca-Cola when it was introduced. Soda sizes have gotten so big that auto manufacturers have installed larger cup holders to accommodate them.

But it's not just fast-food items that have blimped out over the past few generations. Muffin tins, restaurant dinner plates, and pizza pans are larger, according to studies by Lisa Young, Ph.D., R.D., a nutrition researcher at New York University. Young found that even cookbooks suggest larger portion sizes than in the past. For example, in a 1960s version of *Joy of Cooking,* a brownie recipe was described as yielding 30 pieces, Young says, "but now the exact same recipe tells you to cut it into 16 brownies."

Much of this growth appears to have happened without the

public noticing. In a survey conducted by the nonprofit American Institute for Cancer Research, 62 percent of the respondents said restaurant portions today are the same or smaller than they were a decade ago. But it's more important than ever to pay attention. If you've had a muffin for breakfast every day for years, you may now be starting your day, unwittingly, with twice or three times as many calories as you used to. In her research, Young found one popular brand of muffin to contain nearly 1,000 calories.

And if you're following any of the food pyramids, take note that the U.S. Department of Agriculture has a very different definition of the term "serving" than do most restaurants and food manufacturers. For example, a USDA standard meat serving is 2 to 3 ounces, and the maximum recommendation is two to three servings per day. However, restaurant steaks generally range from 8 ounces to 24 ounces; in other words, the steak you order at Bubba's BBQ may contain 12 servings by U.S. government standards. According to Young's research, today's cookies are, on average, 700 percent larger than the USDA standards, and restaurant pasta servings exceed the government's standards by 480 percent.

What's driving this trend? For one thing, food companies have greater profit margins on larger items, so they have an incentive to serve you more. It costs them just pennies more to super-size that soda or movie popcorn, yet they can charge a bundle extra. Savvy marketing tactics play a role, too. Food suppliers long ago determined that customers are typically embarrassed to buy two servings of an item but are willing to buy a single item that's twice as big.

Compounding the problem, value-conscious Americans simply demand larger portions. Jumbo sizes often seem like a bargain. For instance, 7-Eleven's 16-ounce Gulp costs just under 5 cents per ounce, whereas a 32-ounce Big Gulp costs just 2.7 cents per ounce. But in truth, it's the vendors who may be getting the best deal of all. Interestingly, American fast-food franchises offer smaller portions in Europe. McDonald's "extra large" soda portions in London and Rome are the same as the U.S. "large." "Portions in Europe are growing," Young says, "but they're still way behind us. The customers there just don't want it."

Still, there's hope for Americans: Kraft Foods, makers of Oreos, Mallomars, and Chips Ahoy cookies, recently announced it plans to fight obesity by, among other things, reducing its portion sizes, and, of course, McDonald's has phased out its super-sized fries. Other companies are likely to follow, in large part to protect themselves from lawsuits that blame them for their patrons' obesity.

## Question #92: If I'm trying to lose weight, what's the maximum amount of fat I should eat each day?

*The short answer:* Although researchers are still debating this issue in scientific journals and diet gurus continue to duke it out on the bestseller lists, plenty of evidence suggests that it doesn't especially matter how much fat you eat. Where weight loss is concerned, what really matters is your calorie intake.

*One argument in favor* of limiting dietary fat is that high-fat foods tend to be high in calories. One gram of fat contains 9 calories, whereas a gram of carbohydrate or protein contains just 4 calories. A tablespoon of peanut butter (which is very high in fat) contains about 95 calories, whereas a tablespoon of jam (very low in fat) contains about half that. So if you choose foods low in fat, the theory goes, you're bound to save calories.

But in practice, it isn't clear whether limiting fat grams translates into better calorie control. Fat consumption in the United States has declined over the last 25 years, yet obesity rates have risen. In trials lasting more than a year, the percentage of calories from fat — whether it's 18 percent or 40 percent — seems to make little, if any, difference in weight loss. What appears to matter most for long-term weight control is how many calories you eat relative to how many calories you burn.

## Question #93: Is a low-fat diet the healthiest way to eat?

*The short answer:* Your *total* fat intake has little, if any, bearing on your risk for heart disease and diabetes. The real culprits are the artery-clogging fats, namely saturated and trans fats, found in many animal products and processed foods. Unsaturated fats, including the fats in olive and peanut oils, actually promote heart health.

*For years,* the mantra repeated by many nutritionists and health organizations was: "Don't exceed 30 percent of calories from fat." But in recent years, many nutrition experts have backed away from that figure. Instead, the message has become: Choose heart-healthy fats and limit saturated and trans fats to no more than 10 percent of total calories.

How do we know that total fat consumption doesn't matter? The classic evidence is the traditional Mediterranean diet. People who followed this diet, such as residents of the Greek island of Crete circa 1960, got 40 percent of their calories from fat, yet their heart-disease rates were among the lowest in the world. This was in large part because the fat they consumed was almost entirely unsaturated fat from olive oil and fish. At the same time, heart-disease rates were 15 times higher in eastern Finland; total fat consumption was about 38 percent, but the majority of it was saturated fats from meat and dairy products. Even followers of the traditional Japanese diet, consisting of just 10 percent fat, had heart-disease rates more than twice as high as those of the residents of Crete.

More recent studies have bolstered the notion that not only do some fats clog arteries, but other fats actually protect the heart. Research has shown that diets in which about 35 percent of calories come from monounsaturated fat, primarily olive oil, may actually do a better job of reducing heart-disease risk than the low-fat (25 percent fat) diet traditionally recommended for that purpose.

Saturated fat is the artery-clogging variety found primarily in animal products, such as beef, chicken, milk, and cheese. Trans fats, found in fried foods and processed baked goods, are equally, if not more, damaging to the arteries. They're created through hydrogenation, a process that turns liquid oils into solids, making pie crusts flakier and French fries crispier.

As of 2006, the U.S. government will require trans fat informa-

## More Artery-Clogging Fat Than Meets the Eye

As this chart indicates, saturated fat accounts for only half the artery-clogging fat contained in many processed foods. Now that trans fat will be listed on food labels, the public will have a more accurate idea of just how unhealthy many foods are. Your combined percentage of saturated and trans fat should not exceed 10 percent of your total caloric intake.

### Total Fat, Saturated Fat, and Trans Fat Content per Serving (Grams)

| Product | Common Serving Size | Total Fat | Saturated Fat | Trans Fat | Combined Sat & Trans Fats |
|---|---|---|---|---|---|
| French fried potatoes (fast food) ± | Medium size | 26.9 | 6.7 | 7.8 | **14.5** |
| Butter | 1 tbsp | 10.8 | 7.2 | 0.3 | **7.5** |
| Margarine (stick) † | 1 tbsp | 11.0 | 2.1 | 2.8 | **4.9** |
| Margarine (tub) † | 1 tbsp | 6.7 | 1.2 | 0.6 | **1.8** |
| Mayonnaise (soybean oil) ‡ | 1 tbsp | 10.8 | 1.6 | 0.0 | **1.6** |
| Shortening ± | 1 tbsp | 13.0 | 3.4 | 4.2 | **7.6** |
| Potato chips ± | Small bag | 11.2 | 1.9 | 3.2 | **5.1** |
| Milk (whole) ± | 1 cup | 6.6 | 4.3 | 0.2 | **4.5** |
| Doughnut ± | 1 | 18.2 | 4.7 | 5.0 | **9.7** |
| Cookies (cream filled) ± | 3 | 6.1 | 1.2 | 1.9 | **3.1** |
| Cake (pound) ± | 1 slice | 16.4 | 3.4 | 4.3 | **7.7** |

† Values derived from 2002 USDA National Nutrient Database for Standard Reference, Release 15.
‡ Prerelease values derived from 2002 USDA National Nutrient Database for Standard Reference, Release 16.
± 1995 USDA composition data.

tion to be included on food labels, enabling the public to finally see that many foods are twice as harmful as they previously appeared. For instance, a large order of Burger King onion rings contains 7 grams of trans fat, in addition to the 6 listed grams of saturated fat shown on the BK Web site. That's 13 grams of artery-clogging fat in one side order — more than half the daily limit of unhealthy fat recommended by most health organizations. If you eat 2,000 calories a day, you should limit your combined intake of saturated and trans fats to about 22 grams (10 percent of total calories).

## Question #94: What is a low-carb diet?

*The short answer:* It depends on whom you ask.

*The U.S. Department of Agriculture* recommends getting at least 55 percent of your calories from carbohydrates, preferably from high-fiber, nutrient-rich sources such as whole grains, fruits, and vegetables. This government agency refers to any eating plan below 55 percent carbohydrates as "low-carb." (The FDA will soon be issuing its own definition of "low-carb" for food-labeling purposes.) On the other hand, diets such as the Zone, which advises getting 40 percent of your total caloric intake from carbs, adamantly claim not to be low-carb. After all, Zone proponents point out, you're still getting nearly half your calories from carbohydrates.

Eating plans like the Atkins Diet are decidedly low-carb by any definition. During your first two weeks on Atkins, the so-called "induction phase," you're allowed only about 5 percent of your calories from carbs, which equates to about 20 grams of carbs or a ½ cup of pasta. After two weeks of dieting, you're permitted 10 to 15 percent of your calories from carbs, roughly 40 to 60 grams

## The Lowdown on Low-Carb Diets

| Popular Diet Program | % Carb Calories | % Protein Calories | % Fat Calories | % Sat fat Calories | Cholesterol (mg) | Fiber (grams) |
|---|---|---|---|---|---|---|
| Atkins | 5–15 | 35 | 59 | 26 | 924 | 4 |
| Protein Power | 8 | 35 | 53 | 19 | 657 | 11 |
| Sugar Busters! | 40 | 28 | 32 | 9 | 280 | 24 |
| The Zone | 32 | 28 | 32 | 7 | 264 | 18 |
| Ornish | 74 | 18 | 7 | 2 | 30 | 49 |
| U.S. government recommendations | 55–58 | 12 | 30 | 10 (max) | <300 | 25–35 |

of carbs and equivalent to about 1¼ cups of rice or 4 slices of bread. This diet is not only low in carbs but it's also high in fat, much of it saturated fat from animal-based and full-fat dairy products.

When a low-carb diet is referenced as part of a research study, it usually means that subjects were limited to about 40 grams of carbs a day. A "very-low-carb" diet usually refers to a daily limit of 20 to 25 grams of carbs.

What the difference between a high-protein and a low-carb diet? It's largely a matter of semantics, though low-carb proponents say that the whole point is to eat fewer carbs, not more protein per se. They say these diets are higher in protein — and often higher in fat — because you've got to replace the missing carbs with something.

## Question #95: Are low-carb, high-protein diets safe?

*The short answer:* In the short term, yes. In the long run, who knows?

*For decades experts* have warned against low-carb diets, fearing they would cause an epidemic of hardened arteries, skyrocketing cholesterol levels, and rapidly disintegrating bone mass. Well, this is one case where the experts appear to be wrong — at least in the short term.

Several prominent investigations, including two conducted at Harvard University, found that dieters who ate an abundance of protein and saturated fats while restricting grains and other plant-based foods actually improved their cholesterol profiles to a greater extent than those who followed the kind of low-fat diet recommended by the American Heart Association. Not only that, in these studies — conducted on obese subjects — low-carbers lost nearly twice as much weight as low-fat dieters without suffering any immediately increased risk of stroke or decreased bone density. (However, as we explain in Question #96, neither group lost a whole lot of weight, and after a year, the low-carbers had re-gained weight and were no slimmer than the low-fat dieters.)

One well-established and immediate consequence of eating a low-carb diet is the formation of ketones, chemicals created when there is not enough insulin in the blood and your body must break down fat for energy. For most people this occurs when they dip below 50 grams of carbs per day over a significant period of time. This "ketosis" process can cause nausea, lightheadedness, and bad breath. Most low-carb dieters report some mild discomfort and unpleasantness brought on by ketosis for a few weeks.

Bad breath and upset tummies aside, it appears your body won't fall apart from a few months of low-carb dieting. However, decades of research indicate that eating more than two to three times the level of U.S. dietary recommendations for protein on a regular basis increases the level of urinary calcium, which many experts believe is a sign of bone mass being slowly leached away. It may also signal an increased risk of developing kidney prob-lems, particularly kidney stones. And any diet that skimps on whole grains, fruits, and veggies lacks important vitamins, miner-als, and other essential nutrients. Many experts think that over a period of time, this increases risk for cancer and cardiac disease as well as liver, kidney, and bone diseases.

Still, no study has examined the safety of low-carb eating be-yond a year. Many of the potential long-range risks are being in-ferred from studies that looked at diet in combination with a host of other health and lifestyle factors such as exercise, smoking, and stress. These studies certainly point to a high consumption of meat and saturated fat as an unhealthy behavior that leads to serious, chronic health problems. A definitive answer requires controlled, long-duration studies that isolate dietary factors from other health habits. To date, no such study exists on low-carb dieting.

So for now, if you're planning a lifetime of high-protein, low-carb menus, proceed with caution. Currently, most experts, even low-carb proponents, don't recommend this kind of diet for any-one with an existing kidney condition, a predisposition for kidney problems, or diabetes.

## Question #96: Are low-carb diets effective for weight loss?

*The short answer:* Although preliminary research suggests that obese people can initially lose more weight on a low-carb diet than on a conventional low-fat diet, the benefits appear to be small and may be short-lived. The only study lasting a full year found that low-carb dieters began regaining weight after six months; by the end of the year, the low-carbers were no better off than the low-fat group. What's more, the dropout rate among both groups was extremely high.

*"Atkins Vindicated!"* "Low-Carb Diets More Effective!" Headlines like these continue to dominate the media. When two Harvard University studies published in the *New England Journal of Medicine* found that obese subjects on a diet touted by Robert Atkins, M.D., the late low-carb guru, lost more weight than dieters who followed a low-fat plan, it was big news worldwide. But did these studies truly prove Atkins right or were the headlines an exaggeration?

In Atkins's favor, the Harvard studies do seem to suggest that, despite prior warnings from health organizations, low-carb diets (defined in Question #94) are safe — at least in the short term. But before you replace that apple a day with eggs and bacon, you should know what most media outlets didn't bother to report — or buried in their stories: About 40 percent of the dieters in both the low-carb and low-fat groups dropped out of the study. What's more, the amount of weight loss among both groups was relatively small. The low-carbers who stuck with the program in the six-month study lost about 12.8 pounds, compared with 4.2 pounds dropped by the low-fat group. Given both groups' relative obesity — the average subject weighed about 286 pounds — that's a drop in the bucket. Even less impressive, the one-year study reported that the weight-loss difference between the two groups was too small to count.

And if the Atkins diet is truly a pound-melting panacea, then why are Americans getting fatter? Since 1972, more than 15 million copies of Atkins's books have been sold. Yet the National Weight Control Registry, a survey of more than 3,000 people who successfully lost at least 30 pounds and kept them off for more than a year, reported that less than 1 percent of participants lost their weight by following a high-protein diet. If subsisting on hamburgers truly offered some sort of metabolic advantage for weight loss, surely the diet would be better represented.

### Question #97: Why do low-carb diets seem to be effective in the short run?

*The short answer:* Initially, low-carb diets promote greater water loss than low-fat diets. They may also be more satisfying and easier to stick with. But in the long run, the advantages don't seem to hold up.

*Restricting carbs* does seem to provide a weight-loss edge in the early days of a diet. To understand why requires a quick and easy chemistry lesson. Carbs are stored in the muscles as glycogen, which is made of thousands of sugar molecules. Glycogen is big and bulky and naturally attracts water into your muscles. When you eat a diet that's high in protein and low in carbs, you diminish your glycogen stores, which in turn causes you to shed water. (Depleted glycogen is why you immediately feel less bloated but also more sluggish during the first week or so of a low-carb plan.)

In fact, this is exactly what a University of Cincinnati study found when comparing a low-fat diet group to a low-carb diet group. Over the course of six months, the low-fat group lost 5 pounds and the low-carb group lost 10 pounds. But 40 percent of the weight that was dropped — 3.5 pounds for the low-fat group and 7 pounds for the low-carb group — was lost in the first two weeks. The researchers attributed the majority of both groups' early losses to water.

But not all of the weight-loss differences between low-fat and low-carb eating can be explained away by water loss. In most studies, about 60 percent of the weight lost from any type of diet is fat (the rest is water and muscle). One theory is that restricting carbs and consuming a lot of protein is more satisfying than limiting fat, so high-protein eaters eat less because they feel fuller for longer. Indeed, several studies show that low-carb dieters report feeling fuller than those on a low-fat plan. It's also possible that the restrictive nature of many low-carb plans may help dieters adhere to them. With fewer choices, it may be easier to limit your calorie intake.

Another theory currently under investigation is that high-protein diets may somehow give your metabolism a slight boost or that you may burn up more energy digesting protein than carbs or fat. Intriguing, but researchers simply don't know yet whether this is true. It could be that the meat eaters in various studies exercised more or misreported their calorie counts. Researchers don't discount these possibilities, but these measures are difficult to track and quantify.

Whatever the reasons for low-carb eating's early advantages, they don't seem to last. Inevitably, most people slowly return to their original eating habits and regain at least half of their weight loss within two years regardless of what type of diet they are on. Based on the information gathered to this point, you shouldn't expect your long-term success to be any greater on a low-carb diet plan than with any other type of eating strategy.

## Question #98: Do I need more protein if I exercise?

*The short answer:* Yes, but not as much extra protein as you might have heard and not enough to require taking protein supplements. Most people who exercise, even serious endurance and strength athletes, easily meet — and typically exceed — their protein needs through their daily meals and snacks.

*Although the claims* on protein-supplement packages tend to be overblown, there is some truth to the notion that serious exercisers, especially weightlifters and endurance athletes, need extra protein. This isn't because protein builds muscles. Exercise — not Ripped Fuel Protein Drink — is what beefs up your quads, glutes, and delts. However, strength training damages muscle cells and a certain amount of protein is required to repair them.

Additional protein is important for marathon runners, distance cyclists, and other endurance athletes because prolonged moderate- to high-intensity aerobic exercise uses a small amount of protein as fuel. (The vast majority of the energy — probably about 90 percent — comes from carbohydrate and fat.) Also, aerobic exercise increases the amounts of certain proteins in the body, including some enzymes and hemoglobin, a protein carried by red cells. So an aerobic exercise enthusiast may need extra dietary protein to help build and maintain these new proteins.

Just how much extra protein does a dedicated exerciser need?

## Where to Get Your Protein

Here's a rundown of some nutritious sources of protein, both vegetarian and non-vegetarian.

| Food | Serving Size | Grams of Protein | Total Calories |
|------|--------------|------------------|----------------|
| Turkey breast, no skin | 4 oz. | 34.0 | 153 |
| Beef, roast, no visible fat | 4 oz. | 33.3 | 272 |
| Tuna in water | 4 oz. | 31.7 | 144 |
| Fish, haddock | 4 oz. | 21.0 | 105 |
| Chicken breast, no skin | 4 oz. | 35.6 | 189 |
| Eggs | 1 | 6.2 | 79 |
| Yogurt, plain, low fat | 1 cup | 11.9 | 143 |
| Milk, skim | 1 cup | 8.3 | 86 |
| Cheese, American | 1 slice | 6.3 | 106 |
| Soybeans, cooked | ½ cup | 9.9 | 117 |
| Tofu | ½ cup | 9.8 | 90 |
| Chickpeas, cooked | ½ cup | 8.4 | 133 |
| Lentils, cooked | ½ cup | 7.8 | 106 |
| Kidney beans, cooked | ½ cup | 7.3 | 114 |
| Peanut butter | 1 tbsp | 3.9 | 87 |
| Oatmeal | 1 cup | 6.0 | 145 |

About 50 to 100 percent more than the Recommended Daily Allowance. The RDA for protein is .36 grams per pound of body weight — about 50 grams of protein daily for a 150-pound person who consumes 2,000 calories. This is the amount considered sufficient to provide the amino acids needed to build and repair red blood cells, enzymes, and other tissues in the body. Consistent exercisers, research suggests, should consume protein in the range of .55 to .8 grams per pound of body weight; that's about 83 to 120 grams of protein for our 150-pound sample person. There's no evidence that exceeding .9 grams of protein (135 grams per day) per pound of body weight will provide any benefit, even for someone auditioning for sequels to *The Hulk*. There is, however, evidence that consuming more than twice the recommended protein intake may increase your risk of kidney and liver problems, and perhaps bone-density loss.

To give you an idea of how easy it is to meet even the upper ranges of these protein recommendations, consider that a chicken Burrito Mexicano at the popular national chain Baja Fresh contains 51 grams of protein, primarily from the chicken and beans. If you round out your day with a bowl of Special K (6 grams) with a cup of milk (9 grams) for breakfast and a turkey breast sandwich (25 grams, including two slices of bread) with a side of cottage cheese (15 grams per half cup) for lunch, you're already at 106 grams of protein for the day, and that doesn't even count snacks or other side dishes.

If you're a vegetarian, getting protein takes a bit more work, but there are plenty of nutritious plant sources of protein, including beans (about 15 grams per cup), tofu (10 grams per ½ cup), hummus (6 grams per ½ cup), and peanut butter (about 4 grams per tablespoon).

## Question #99: Could fast food really be addictive?

*The short answer:* Perhaps. Some research suggests that foods high in fat and calories may be addictive, at least in rats.

*In 2002 Caesar Barber,* a 56-year-old diabetic and two-time heart-attack victim, filed suit against McDonald's, Burger King, Wendy's, and KFC, claiming that his illnesses were partly their fault. He'd eaten in their establishments for years, he maintained, without ever being warned that their food could harm his health. On the face of it, the case sounded bogus. Surely it's no secret that a Whopper is not health food. Barber seemed to be using the legal system to compensate for his own lack of control and common sense.

Still, there may be a kernel of truth to Barber's argument — or at least to the notion that he wasn't entirely responsible for his plight. Maybe Barber couldn't control his fat cravings because he was actually addicted to fast food. Research suggests the idea isn't entirely preposterous.

For instance, studies on rats suggest the brain can become hard-wired to crave a hit of extra-crispy chicken, just as it might any addictive substance. In a trial conducted at Albert Einstein College of Medicine in New York City, rats fed a diet similar in composition to the typical fast-food meal — that is, high in calories and fat — were less able to respond to leptin, a hormone that signals the hypothalamus gland to regulate eating behavior and signal fullness. (Question #81 explains more about leptin.) Chowing down on fatty foods sent the rats' leptin levels soaring, but their hypothalamuses didn't register the increase, so the rats continued to eat. When the rats were put on a diet and forced to lose weight, subsequent dips in leptin sent their brains the mixed-up signal that they were in danger of starvation, causing them to overeat.

The inappropriate leptin response kicked in after the rats ate just a few high-fat meals, researchers found. Within 72 hours, the rats lost almost all their ability to respond to leptin. The fatter the rats become, scientists speculate, the more resistant they become to leptin's effects, and the harder it is to reverse the trend.

Of course, a rat is not a person any more than a laboratory is a fast-food joint. The biological processes of eating and hunger are complex. They're governed by more than a single hormone and, at least for us humans, convoluted by a host of psychological and social factors. Although most of the leptin studies have been conducted on rats, some research does suggest a similar response in humans.

Not surprisingly, Barber's case was dismissed for lack of merit. His legal strategy was modeled after suits brought against the tobacco industry, but whereas the addictive properties of tobacco are clear, burger-and-fries dependency is still in question.

## Question #100: Can fiber help me lose weight?

*The short answer:* Quite likely.

*If you're trying to shed pounds* and improve your health, chances are you're aiming to cut back — on calories, on sugar, on processed foods, on fried foods, on saturated fat. But when it comes to fiber, your approach should be just the opposite: more, more, more. The typical American consumes about 15 grams of fiber per day — significantly less than the 25 grams to 38 grams recommended by major health organizations for women and men, respectively. Increasing your fiber intake to meet that recommendation not only may reduce your risk of developing colon cancer but may be just the ticket to controlling your weight.

Fiber is a catchall term for indigestible substances found only in plant foods. Fiber comes in two varieties: insoluble and soluble. Insoluble fiber is best known for keeping you "regular"; it holds on to water, helping move waste through the body. Insoluble fiber is found in fruits, vegetables, dried beans, wheat bran, seeds, popcorn, and whole-grain breads and cereals. Soluble fiber — the type shown to reduce blood-cholesterol levels — is found in oats, peas, beans, barley, rye, and several fruits.

Both types of fiber are valuable for weight control. High-fiber foods tend to be low in calories, so you can pile your plate full without piling on calories. A heaping salad of spinach, carrots, zucchini, broccoli, onion, tomato, three-bean salad, and low-calorie dressing contains about 150 calories — less than a small Coke at Burger King. Fiber-rich foods also tend to require more chewing than foods void of fiber, so your brain has time to register full-ness before you've overeaten. Think about how long it takes to eat an apple (3 grams of fiber) compared with gulping a 6-ounce glass of apple juice (no fiber), and think about which leaves you feeling more full.

In studies where people are allowed to eat as much as they want, subjects given high-fiber meals consume about 10 percent fewer calories than people served foods lower in fiber. The effect seems to be greatest with overweight people. A review of several studies found that, when given high-fiber foods, overweight or obese people ate, on average, 18 percent fewer calories than over-weight people offered low-fiber foods.

To increase your fiber intake, eat whole fruits instead of fruit juices and choose whole-grain breads and cereals. Just make sure you read food labels carefully and look for "whole wheat" instead of "wheat." A bread called "12 grain" might be 90 percent white flour dressed up with caramel coloring and a few sprinkles of grains and contain the same amount of fiber — 1 gram — as a slice of plain white Wonder Bread.

## Question #101: Will artificial sweeteners help me lose weight?

*The short answer:* In theory, yes. Drinking diet sodas and aspar-tame-sweetened yogurts will save you lots of calories, but there's conflicting research on whether using these products actually helps with weight control.

*It seems like a no-brainer:* Switch from regular Coke (150 calo-ries) to Diet Coke (zero calories) and you'll shed pounds. But con-sider this: The United States leads the world in consumption of artificial sweeteners, yet we are also one of the world's fattest na-tions. The dramatic increase in artificially sweetened products on the market — some 6,000 products are now sweetened with as-partame (first introduced in 1981) — has coincided with a dra-matic increase in obesity rates (see Question #3).

Would we be an even fatter nation without these products? Who knows? The reasons for the skyrocketing obesity rates are complex and numerous. However, there's also little reason to believe that the introduction of artificially sweetened products, which generally contain far fewer calories than their naturally sweetened counterparts, has helped control our girth.

In the scientific community, there's no consensus as to whether artificial sweeteners help with weight control. Most of the published studies have been short-term, lasting just a few hours to a few days. In some studies, subjects served artificially sweetened foods and drinks ate fewer calories over the course of the day than those who consumed naturally sweetened products. Other studies found just the opposite; researchers speculated that diet foods and drinks might be less satisfying, subconsciously leading people to compensate by consuming more food later on. Only one trial lasted as long as 10 weeks. In that study, the group served diet products lost on average 2.2 pounds (mostly water weight), whereas the group served sugar-sweetened foods and drinks gained 3.5 pounds.

If you choose artificially sweetened products, keep in mind that they're no free ticket to weight loss. Pay close attention to calories you're eating and drinking when you're *not* downing that Diet Sprite or Yoplait Light.

## Question #102: What is the glycemic index, and is it important for weight loss?

*The short answer:* The glycemic index (GI) is a ranking of foods on a scale of 0 to 100, based on how much they spike blood-sugar levels right after you eat. Foods with a low glycemic index tend to be more satisfying than high-GI foods, so they may help you control your calorie intake. However, the glycemic index isn't a weight-loss silver bullet, and there are times when high-GI foods are a better choice.

*Carbs may not be the evildoers* some pop nutritionists would have you believe, but which carbs you choose may make a difference when you're trying to lose weight. One reason is that carbs differ in their score on the glycemic index.

Glucose, which is pure sugar, is the most quickly digested form of carbohydrate, and it scores 100 on the GI. All other foods are given a number relative to glucose. Foods with a high GI score, such as corn flakes (84) and vanilla wafers (77), are rapidly digested and absorbed into the bloodstream. They tend to be high in refined sugars, low in soluble fiber, highly processed, soft, or extremely ripe. Low-GI foods — for instance, soybeans (18) and grapefruits (25) — are more slowly digested and absorbed, so they produce a more gradual rise in blood sugar and insulin. Foods with a GI of 70 or more are considered high-GI; foods that rate less than 55 are considered low-GI; anything in between is considered to have a moderate GI.

Studies suggest that eating a diet packed with low-GI foods may help tame your appetite because these foods are more satisfying. That's why you may feel ravenous a few hours after eating a couple of pieces of toast with jam, whereas a bowl of old-fashioned oatmeal with nuts can keep you going until lunch. Although these two meals might contain roughly the same number of calories, the lower GI rating of the oatmeal may make all the difference in your satiety level.

Other studies show that high-GI foods stimulate your appetite by causing insulin spikes that ultimately send your blood-sugar levels crashing. Still other research suggests that eating low-GI foods may improve endurance during cardio activities and perhaps help you avoid or control Type 2 diabetes and fend off heart disease and some forms of cancer.

But keep in mind that you can't simply choose carbs with the lowest GI and expect pounds to drop off. Counting calories and limiting portions will always be the most important part of any weight-loss plan. Also, you can blunt the effects of high-GI foods to some extent by combining them with low-GI foods and foods high in fiber, fat, or protein. A slice of high-GI bread topped with low-GI peanut butter is absorbed more slowly than a slice of the bread alone. To find a food's GI and decide which foods to combine for a more desirable GI effect, refer to a database such as the one found at glycemicindex.com.

But before you judge a food solely by its GI, know that the *amount* of carbohydrate in a food also makes a difference in the impact it has on your blood sugar. Carrots, for example, have a high GI (92) but contain just 5 grams of carbs per ½ cup. This makes a carrot's impact on your blood sugar (often referred to as "glycemic load") minimal compared with that of instant rice, which has a GI of 91 but a substantial 18 grams of carbs per ½-cup serving.

That said, there may be times you want to go high-GI. Many high-GI foods, like unpeeled carrots and potatoes, supply a wealth of nutrients. And many breakfast cereals, like Cheerios (GI = 74) and bran flakes (GI = 74), are fortified with vitamins and minerals and supply a good dose of heart-healthy fiber.

Eating high-GI foods and beverages during and after exercise also helps boost performance and recovery. Sports drinks and energy bars (both high-GI) can deliver an immediate source of sugar to your working muscles. After exercise, high-GI foods work best to replenish glycogen stores.

## Question #103: What exactly is cholesterol?

*The short answer:* It's a waxy substance made in your liver and contained in animal foods such as meat, poultry, and dairy products. High blood cholesterol leads to clogged arteries, but your body does need some cholesterol to insulate nerves, promote healthy cell growth, and produce certain hormones.

*Cholesterol* attaches itself to substances known as lipoproteins. Like microscopic taxi drivers, lipoproteins shuttle cholesterol molecules through the bloodstream from place to place.

Some lipoproteins — low-density lipoproteins, a.k.a. LDL — are responsible for delivering cholesterol to the cells. Another type — high-density lipoproteins, known as HDL — are responsible for picking up and disposing of excess amounts. Sometimes the LDL doesn't make it to its destination and instead sticks to the walls of your arteries. If you don't have enough HDL cholesterol to scrub your arteries clean, LDL builds up, clogging your blood vessels like too much sludge in a drain and increasing your risk for developing atherosclerosis (hardening of the arteries). That's why HDL is considered the "good" cholesterol and LDL is known as the "bad" kind. A third group of carrier molecules, very-low-density lipoproteins (VLDL), are converted to LDL after distributing triglycerides to the muscles and fat tissue.

A combined cholesterol level (HDL, LDL, and VLDL) of less than 200 after at least eight hours of fasting is considered ideal. People who have a total cholesterol level of 275 or greater are at significantly increased risk for developing coronary problems, even if their HDL levels are favorable. People who have normal cholesterol levels but low HDL levels are also at increased risk for a heart attack. More than half of all Americans have higher-than-recommended cholesterol levels, and high cholesterol is a leading risk factor for heart disease. See the chart on page 142 for current American Heart Association cholesterol guidelines.

Like many health problems, high cholesterol comes from a combination of genetics and poor lifestyle habits. Men tend to have higher LDL levels and lower HDL levels than do premenopausal women. Once women hit menopause, their decreasing levels of estrogen correspond with declining HDLs and increased risk for heart disease.

Losing weight, eating a diet low in saturated fat, quitting smoking, and reducing stress can all potentially help decrease LDLs and

## Cholesterol Levels: How High Is Too High?

|  | Desirable | Borderline | Undesirable |
|---|---|---|---|
| Total Cholesterol | Below 200 | 200–240 | Above 240 |
| HDL Cholesterol | Above 45 | 35–45 | Below 35 |
| LDL Cholesterol | Below 130 | 130–160 | Above 160 |
| Total Cholesterol/HDL | Below 4.5 | 4.5–5.5 | Above 5.5 |

increase HDLs. Interestingly, foods high in cholesterol don't raise blood-cholesterol levels as much as foods high in saturated fat. Consuming monounsaturated fats such as olive oil and peanuts may also reduce LDL levels. For people with very high cholesterol levels or levels that don't seem to budge with lifestyle changes, doctors often prescribe cholesterol-lowering drugs.

## Question #104: Will drinking lots of water help me lose weight?

*The short answer:* Probably not, although the topic isn't well studied.

*Many people assume* that water helps with weight loss by making you feel full. The more water you drink, the theory goes, the fewer calories you eat. But actually, a number of studies suggest otherwise.

For example, University of Pennsylvania researchers examined how drinking water affects calorie consumption by comparing three groups of women. One group was offered a chicken-and-rice casserole, a second group ate the same casserole and downed a large glass of water, and the other ate a bowl of chicken soup containing roughly the same number of calories as the casserole. Both chicken casserole–eating groups reported the same level of satisfaction and ate approximately the same number of calories in later meals. Drinking water didn't seem to have any calorie-reducing advantage at all.

But interestingly, the soup eaters reported feeling the most satisfied and consequently ate about one-third fewer calories than the other two groups. This led the researchers to speculate that drinking water with a meal doesn't fill you up or leave you feeling any more satisfied than passing on the water pitcher, but watery foods may, for unknown reasons, leave you feeling more satiated than drinking water with your meals.

Several other studies have found that water does not increase satiety, and neither does it cause water drinkers to consume fewer calories. However, people often mistake thirst for hunger, turning to food when all they really need is a glass of water. So for that reason, staying well hydrated may help with calorie control.

Weight control aside, there are plenty of important reasons to maintain a consistent fluid intake. Your body is a virtual planet Earth; it's nearly 70 percent water. You lose water during various biological functions, such as breathing, perspiring, and going to the bathroom. Taking in adequate amounts of water keeps your skin healthy, your brain functioning properly, and your blood flowing freely.

How much water is enough? The conventional wisdom is to drink at least eight 8-ounce glasses of water daily, but the origin of this rule is somewhat of a mystery. The Institute of Medicine of the National Academies, a group of scientists who study food recommendations for accuracy, recently concluded that most people meet their daily hydration needs simply by letting thirst be their guide. Exercisers, of course, need more than inactive people (see Question #105 for details), and those who live in hot or cold climates or at high altitudes also need more water than the average person. Keep in mind that there are many ways to hydrate. About 20 percent of the water you take in daily is likely to come from foods, including fruits and vegetables.

In general, it appears that adults have built-in mechanisms such as thirst and sweat to signal when we should drink water, so the best advice is simply to listen to your body.

## Question #105: How much water should I drink when I work out?

*The short answer:* The answer depends on how much you sweat, but in general sipping 8 to 12 ounces every 20 minutes or so should keep you well hydrated.

*Many health books* and Internet sites offer fairly alarmist advice about fluid needs during exercise, recommending that you "drink twice as much as you need to quench your thirst" or "force your-

self to drink every 10 minutes or so even if you don't feel like it."
In truth, while it's important to drink plenty of fluids — to prevent dehydration and to operate at your best — there's no need to
obsess about your fluid intake during exercise.

It's a good idea to wet your whistle at about the same rate you
sweat. For most of us, that's about 8 to 12 ounces of liquid every
20 minutes or so during exercise, more if it's extremely hot or
you're sweating profusely. You're slightly dehydrated if your
mouth and lips feel dry and you feel somewhat thirsty. If you
pinch your skin and there's no spring to it, you're more than
mildly dehydrated and should drink as soon as possible. Dehydration can trigger cramps, zap your stamina, cloud your thinking, and, in very extreme cases, even cause death.

Although exercisers are most obviously prone to dehydration
in hot, humid weather, it's just as important to drink up when
you're working out in cold, dry weather. You may not notice
yourself sweating when you're layered in winter workout gear, especially with all the high-tech winter fabrics that "instantly wick
perspiration off your skin," but rest assured, you're still perspiring. Plus, cold, dry air doesn't hold as much water as warmer air,
so when you breathe, your body extracts water from your tissues
to humidify the air before it gets to your lungs, leaving you more
susceptible to dehydration.

To make sure you've replenished fluids sufficiently, you may
want to weigh yourself before and after your workouts. For every
pound of water you lose during exercise, drink a pint (16 ounces)
of water. If you've been hydrating well enough while you work
out, you'll probably weigh the same or just slightly less afterward.

Studies show that sports drinks and flavored, low-calorie vitamin waters may do a better job of quenching your thirst than
water — probably because they taste good, so you drink more.
Gatorade or any beverage that contains small amounts of sugar
and electrolytes (dissolved sodium and potassium) may keep you
feeling more energetic longer, and such drinks help replace the
electrolytes you lose through sweat. These drinks are probably
best reserved for exercise sessions on hot days that last for more

than an hour or anytime you're doing a really long workout, like a three-hour bike ride. Otherwise the additional electrolytes are probably unnecessary, and you may wind up drinking just as many calories as you burn off.

You probably want to jog right past the juice bar and perhaps the soda machine, too. Full-strength fruit juices may leave you doubled over with cramps, and some people report cramping from carbonation, although this topic hasn't been well studied. Caffeinated beverages such as coffee and tea have a diuretic effect, causing you to shed water at a faster-than-usual rate, so they may not be the best choice.

Although sports nutrition experts have long cautioned exercisers about dehydration, recently they have begun to warn that guzzling too much water is just as dangerous as being parched. This concern has resulted in several respected organizations revising their fluid intake recommendations to include upper as well as lower limits. For instance, not long ago, USA Track & Field, the national governing body for track and field, long-distance running, and race walking, issued an advisory warning athletes that drinking too much can cause hyponatremia, a condition whereby the blood is so diluted that the concentration of sodium plummets. Though relatively rare, the incidence of hyponatremia appears to be highest for marathoners, triathletes, long-distance cyclists, and others who exercise for several hours or more in the heat. Symptoms of early hyponatremia include disorientation and cramping. In extreme cases, it can lead to death. The Institute of Medicine of the National Academies is likely to follow USA Track & Field, issuing similar upper-limit fluid intake recommendations.

## Question #106: How long should I wait between my last meal and my workout?

*The short answer:* It's a good idea to wait about two hours between your last full meal and an intense workout; otherwise your stomach is likely to slosh around like the rinse cycle of a washing machine. However, if you've only nibbled on a light snack, you can probably exercise sooner.

*For most people,* two hours seems to be about the right amount of time between a full meal and full workout to prevent feelings of sluggishness and nausea. Try to avoid greasy foods as part of your last pre-exercise meal, as they're more likely to sit in your stomach. Wait a bit longer to exercise if your last meal consisted of hefty portions (not that we recommend eating hefty portions).

Of course, there's a lot of individuality to consider. Some people can go for a 10-mile run right after a trip to an all-you-can-eat salad bar while others can't bear to have anything in their stomachs during a brisk walk. You have to experiment to find the ideal timing of your preworkout meals.

If you're too busy to eat a complete meal a few hours before working out, nutritional experts advise eating a snack that combines a carbohydrate with a high glycemic index (see Question #102) and protein about 30 minutes before exercising. This combination will maximize the amount of glucose in your bloodstream and give you a shot of energy without leaving you feeling too full. Good choices include a banana with some peanut butter and crackers with a little bit of low-fat cheese.

## Question #107: How fattening is alcohol?

*The short answer:* It depends on your beverage of choice, how much booze you drink, and whether one hand is buried in a bowl of buttered popcorn while the other is clutching a Bass Ale.

*If you pound down beer after beer* night after night, you may one day glance down and notice that the view to your feet is obscured by a large, protruding gut. They don't call 'em "beer bellies" for nothing. Three 12-ounce beers will cost you about 450 calories (see the chart on page 147 for alcoholic-beverage calorie counts). And that doesn't count the chips, mondo pizza slices, or other

## Think Before You Drink

Here are calorie estimates for several popular alcoholic beverages. Calorie counts may vary among brands.

|  | Serving Size | Calories |
|---|---|---|
| Beer | 12 oz. | 140–145 |
| Dark beer | 12 oz. | 155–160 |
| "Light" beer | 12 oz. | 100 |
| White wine | 5 oz. | 90–100 |
| Red wine | 5 oz. | 105–110 |
| Champagne | 5 oz. | 115–120 |
| Hard liquor, 80-proof | 1.5 oz. | 97 |
| Hard liquor, 94-proof | 1.5 oz. | 115 |
| Gin and tonic | 8 oz. | 155 |
| Bloody Mary | 5 oz. | 125 |
| Margarita | 8 oz. | 300 |
| Martini | 3.5 oz. | 140 |
| Sherry | 2 oz. | 65 |

high-calorie foods that often go hand in hand with beer drinking.

Not that beer is any worse for your waistline than soda. A 12-ounce can of beer actually contains about the same number of calories as a 12-ounce soda. But alcohol loosens your inhibitions and impairs your judgment, so you may be less careful about the food choices you make while imbibing. Plus, as a double whammy, alcohol stimulates appetite.

If you enjoy a brew with your ball game and are watching your weight, you're best off with light beer, which contains about 100 calories per 12 ounces. Nonalcoholic beer weighs in at around 70 calories. Dark ales tend to have about 10 percent more calories than regular beers.

Of course, beer isn't the only form of alcohol that can cause a bulging belly. Probably the worst offenders, calorie-wise, are those mixed drinks that come with little umbrellas. An 8-ounce margarita or daiquiri contains about 300 calories; a 6.8-ounce can of piña colada will set you back 526 calories. (Of course, that's no worse than many of the fancy coffee drinks described in Question #108.)

A 5-ounce glass of wine, which has the same amount of alcohol as a 12-ounce beer, contains 105 to 115 calories (red wine contains slightly more calories than white). A 1.5-ounce shot of hard liquor contains 90 to 115 calories. The higher the proof, the higher the calories.

## Question #108: Just how many calories are in those fancy coffee drinks?

*The short answer:* Depending on what type and size of drink you order, what type of milk you request, and whether you ask for whipped cream, a daily Starbucks habit can run you from about 75 calories up to a seriously jolting 1,035 calories.

*An ordinary cup of black coffee* contains about 5 calories, but when you've got caramel macchiatos, iced caffe lattes, iced blended mochas, and mocha malt Frappuccinos to choose from, who orders a plain old cup of joe anymore? Although it's tempting to discount the calories you get from beverages, some coffee drinks contain more than half the calories you need in an entire day. Add a scone (500 calories) or a slice of coffeecake (630 calories) to your order, and you've consumed virtually a day's worth of calories in one coffee break. You've also far exceeded the maximum amount of artery-clogging fat recommended for one day. (See Question #93 for information about saturated and trans fats.)

To minimize the calorie count and saturated fat content of coffee drinks, request that they be made with nonfat milk and forgo the whipped cream, which adds 100 calories and 6 grams of saturated fat. The chart on page 149 includes calorie and saturated fat information for many popular coffee drinks at Starbucks. Similar beverages at other coffee establishments vary somewhat but are in the same ballpark.

## How Many Calories in Your Coffee?

If your favorite coffee beverage isn't listed here, check out the Starbucks Web site, starbucks.com. All beverages here apply to the "grande" (16-ounce) size. The calorie counts for drinks at other coffee restaurants may vary.

| Beverage | Calories | Saturated Fat (grams) |
|---|---|---|
| **Cappuccino** | | |
| Whole milk | 150 | 5 |
| 2% milk | 140 | 3 |
| Nonfat milk | 100 | 0 |
| Soy milk | 120 | 0 |
| **Caffe Latte** | | |
| Whole milk | 260 | 9 |
| Nonfat milk | 160 | 0 |
| Soy milk | 210 | 1 |
| **Iced Caffe Latte** | | |
| Whole milk | 160 | 5 |
| Nonfat milk | 100 | 0 |
| Soy milk | 120 | 0 |
| **Frappuccino (no whipped cream)** | | |
| Caramel | 280 | 2 |
| Chocolate brownie | 370 | 6 |
| Coffee | 260 | 2 |
| Espresso | 230 | 2 |
| Mocha | 290 | 2 |
| Mocha malt | 430 | 4 |
| **Frappuccino Blended Creme** | | |
| Vanilla | 350 | 1 |
| Chocolate | 400 | 1.5 |
| Toffee Nut | 360 | 1 |
| Chocolate malt | 470 | 3.5 |

## Question #109: Will Slim Fast and other "meal-replacement" shakes really help me lose weight?

*The short answer:* The success rate for most meal-replacement products seems to be a better-guarded secret than the whereabouts of Jimmy Hoffa. However, some studies show that replacing one or more meals a day with a "diet" shake can be an effective way to lose weight, at least for those who need to lose a great deal.

*The next time* you see a commercial featuring the testimonial of a bikini-clad beauty extolling the virtues of some meal-replacement shake plan, get up close to the TV so you can read the small print that flashes across the bottom of the screen. It reads, "Results not typical."

In reality, meal-replacement companies go to great lengths to hide the facts about how many people achieve long-term, meaningful results from using their products. The Slim Fast Web site answers more than two dozen "frequently asked questions," including whether it's safe to drink a Slim Fast shake while breast-feeding and how much fiber their products contain. But nowhere does the site report how likely you are to lose weight and keep it off based on reliable, scientific evidence. This leads skeptics like us to believe that good results are indeed not typical.

Meal-replacement shakes like Slim Fast, Nestlé's Sweet Success, and others are essentially fortified, low-fat, low-calorie milk shakes that come in flavors like Rich Chocolate Royale and Cappuccino Delight. They typically contain about 200 to 250 calories per 11-ounce serving, along with about 5 grams of fiber and 10 grams of protein. The idea is to drink a shake in place of breakfast, lunch, or dinner; some plans call for replacing two meals a day.

Drinking a meal-replacement shake once or twice a day may help you lose weight by reducing your daily calorie intake, but keeping it off will require that you continue using the shakes indefinitely or practice some other form of calorie restriction — something most people find they can't do because they miss the satisfaction of eating food that can be chewed. And because these shakes limit your food options and don't encourage you to learn how to make nutritious food choices, you're likely to return to your old eating habits once you give them up. To "support" their meal-replacement plans, some companies sell other prepackaged foods, snacks, and supplements. If your taste buds don't shrivel up, your bank account certainly will.

That said, some studies show that mildly to moderately obese people who substitute one or more meals a day with a diet shake can lose weight and keep it off for a period of time. The Obesity Research Center at St. Luke's–Roosevelt Hospital in New York surveyed six such studies lasting at least a year and concluded that meal-replacement shake drinkers lost an average of 5 to 6 pounds more than the subjects who stuck with a reduced-calorie diet. Overall, they lost approximately 7 to 8 percent of their body weight, whereas those in the reduced-calorie groups lost approximately 3 to 7 percent of their body weight.

It should be noted that dropout rates were as high as 35 percent in some of the studies, comparable to the dropout rates in many other weight-loss studies and real-life diet attempts. Although most investigations reported dropout rates, they didn't always factor them into their analysis. In other words, the average weight loss reported applied only to the subjects who completed the study. This may paint a rosier picture of your chances of achieving success than is actually true.

## Question #110: Will vitamins give me energy?

*The short answer:* No, because they don't contain calories.

*Given the way vitamins are marketed* — you can buy "Vitamins for Energy!" or a "Super Energy Pack!" or "Alive Energy Formulas!" — you might think that all you need to do is pop a Flintstones multi and you'll be revved up for the day. But in truth, energy can come only from calories, and calories are derived from three sources: fat, protein, and carbohydrate.

Carbs are the source of fuel that's easiest for your body to break down and convert to a usable form of energy. That's why you turn to a Clif Bar instead of a hamburger for quick energy during a workout. There is a large store of carbohydrate, in the form of sugar, coursing through your bloodstream that's readily available for use. If that supply is running low, your body ultimately turns to fat and protein for fuel. Fats offer the most concentrated form of energy — about 9 calories per gram, compared with 4 calories per gram for carbohydrate and protein. Vitamins contain zippo.

So do vitamins play any role in putting pep in your step? Both vitamins and minerals help in the process of converting food energy into a form that your body can use. You may feel fatigued if your body is short on certain vitamins and minerals, such as B vitamins, iron, and magnesium. This scenario is like your body's equivalent of having a malfunctioning spark plug: You may have plenty of gas in the tank, but if all the other parts aren't working properly to convert the gas into energy, your car won't run very well.

Although it's fine to take a multivitamin daily — in fact, the American Medical Association recommends it — don't consume massive doses of supplements in an attempt to correct a vitamin deficiency you think you may have. If you're unusually fatigued, see your doctor. He or she can run tests to determine whether you truly have a deficiency.

## Question #111: Will I gain weight if I chew a lot of gum?

*The short answer:* Yes, if you chew enough gum that contains sugar.

*Obsessive chompers beware:* One piece of Bubble Yum contains 25 calories, as much as 1 Hershey's Kiss or 4 gumdrops. If you kick a pack-a-day habit (5 pieces), you could save 125 empty calories a day — enough to lose 1 pound a month or 12 pounds in a year. (Of course, this calculation assumes that you're not going to replace the gum with food that contains even more calories.) Big

Red, Doublemint, and Juicy Fruit contain 10 calories per stick. If you gnaw on 5 pieces a day, breaking that habit could save you 5 pounds a year.

What about sugarless gums? The calories can still add up, but they're a better choice to satisfy an oral fixation. A piece of Sugarless Bubble Yum contains a hefty 20 calories, but a stick of most sugar-free gums contains just 5 calories.

Just know that the number of calories in your favorite gum may be a mystery. While most sugarless gums have a Nutrition Facts label on each individual pack, most gums with sugar don't. That's because on small items like gum, the government requires labels only on the box, not on each pack. Not all stores display gum in its original box.

# Cardio Exercise: Target Zones, Intervals, and Intensity

When it comes to cardiovascular exercise — the kind that boosts your stamina, strengthens your heart and lungs, and offers, oh, maybe a hundred other benefits — many exercisers fall into one of two categories. On the one hand, there are the die-hards who plan their workouts with scientific zeal, tossing around terms like lactic acid, anaerobic threshold, and VO2 max. And then there are the people who don't want to know much more than: (1) What's the minimum amount of exercise I can get away with? and (2) Does weed-whacking count?

This section should satisfy the curiosity of exercisers on both ends of the spectrum and anyone in between. When it comes to gauging your exercise intensity and assessing your cardio fitness, we explain the simplest possible methods, as well as formulas and testing procedures ideal for people who calculate the impact of their clothing's wind resistance on the time it takes them to run 3.14359 miles. We also answer questions that are likely to interest anyone who regularly breaks a sweat: Why do my toes get numb on the stairclimber? Will I sweat more — or less — as I become more fit? Is there any advantage to exercising backward? For good measure, we also include tidbits of cardio trivia, such as how the elliptical trainer was invented.

## Question #112: What does *aerobic* mean?

*The short answer: Aerobic* means "with air." The term *aerobic exercise,* coined by Dr. Kenneth Cooper, the father of modern fitness, is used to describe activities that require you to pull extra air into your lungs, so that you can get enough oxygen to your muscles to fuel the workout.

*When you exercise* for more than about two minutes, your muscles demand a supply of oxygen, which your lungs extract from the air — hence the huffing and puffing. Typically, to qualify as aerobic, an activity must be repetitive; must involve large muscle groups such as the hips, legs, back, and chest; and must be intense enough to get your heart beating in your target zone (defined in Question #119) for a majority of the workout. Activities such as running, swimming, and cycling are classic examples of aerobic exercise, but we suppose anything that meets the criteria could be considered aerobic, even vacuuming, if your living room is as big as the Vatican.

*Aerobic* is often used interchangeably with *cardiovascular* and *cardiorespiratory,* since aerobic exercise strengthens the heart and lungs. Traditionally, experts believed that exercise had to last for at least 20 continuous minutes in order to provide benefits, but, as we explain in Question #115, recent research indicates that you get about the same health benefits and burn the same number of calories from doing several short bouts of exercise throughout the day as you do from one long session.

Regular aerobic exercise is essential for burning calories, increasing stamina, and reducing your risk of heart disease, high blood pressure, and other conditions.

## Question #113: What does *anaerobic* mean?

*The short answer: Anaerobic* means "without air." *Anaerobic exercise* refers to very short bursts of exercise, like sprints and weightlifting sets, that don't require oxygen to power them.

*Your body stores* one or two minutes' worth of fuel to fire up your muscles, enough for a 100-yard dash, a set of squats, or a brief session punching the heavy bag. Once you use up that energy, it's like running out of gas in a car. You simply can't continue until more fuel — in this case, oxygen — flows into your tank.

Your body also goes into anaerobic mode when you're working so hard that it can't keep up with your muscles' demand for oxygen, like when a marathoner kicks into high gear to break the tape or a skater powers into a triple Lutz at the end of her routine.

Anaerobic exercise builds strength and speed. The major fitness organizations recommend doing two or three days a week of weight training — each set is its own, self-contained anaerobic session — to keep your muscles strong and your bones healthy. No professional group makes a specific recommendation about sprinting activities for the average person because they carry such a high risk of injury. There's really no need to practice all-out mad dashes, unless you're attending football camp, training for a swim meet, or your job requires you to race after criminals or escape from charging bulls.

## Question #114: How much exercise do I really need?

*The short answer:* Though it seems like every academy, institute, society, and association promotes different exercise guidelines, there's actually somewhat of a consensus on how much physical activity it takes to make you a healthier person: 30 minutes a day. Increasing to 60 minutes a day will further cut your risk of developing certain diseases. Still hotly debated among the experts: the amount of movement you need for weight loss or prevention of weight gain.

*In 2003,* the Institute of Medicine of the National Academies, a panel of esteemed scientists and physicians that advises the government, issued a report stating that adults and children should get a minimum of 60 minutes of physical activity each day. The recommendations made the headlines and caused quite a stir: This was twice the minimum amount recommended since 1996 by the U.S. Surgeon General and endorsed by most medical organizations, including the American College of Sports Medicine, the American Heart Association, the Centers for Disease Control, and the National Institutes of Health.

Since many Americans weren't even coming close to meeting the 30-minute recommendation, some experts felt the new guidelines would only discourage the public, setting standards so high that people would simply throw in the towel. But when you take the time to digest both the 30- and 60-minute recommendations, you see that both pieces of advice are really just two different ways of saying the same thing.

On the one hand, the Surgeon General's guideline recommends accumulating 30 minutes of moderate activity on most or all days of the week — a regimen that can cut by 50 percent your risk of developing coronary heart disease, Type 2 diabetes, and some cancers. If possible, the Surgeon General says, build up to 60 minutes a day to reduce your disease risk by another 10 to 15 percent. On the other hand, the Institute of Medicine recommendations state that you'll get optimal health benefits from doing 60 minutes of activity such as brisk walking or moderately intense cycling. The organization notes that 30 minutes of more vigorous activity, like jogging three or four times a week, is just as effective for decreasing disease risk. Both recommendations emphasize that short bouts of exercise and activity scattered throughout the day count toward your total physical activity quotient.

The Surgeon General's office doesn't say 30 minutes is the ideal; it says a half-hour is the minimum. The Institute of Medicine doesn't say that you must do 60 minutes before you get any health benefits; it says that 60 minutes is the optimum. Both statements are true.

Where the 30- and 60-minute camps part company is on the issue of weight loss and prevention of weight gain. The National Institutes of Health scientists concluded that most people need at least an hour of activity on most days of the week just to prevent weight gain and possibly more than that to lose weight. Most other health organizations, in agreement with the Surgeon General, say this isn't necessarily so. They cite studies in which people have lost weight and kept it off by doing much less activity, and they point out that some people never go near a treadmill their entire lives and still maintain a normal weight. Studies on how much exercise you need for weight loss, they maintain, are all over the map, and individual weight loss depends on what type of activity you do, how much you eat, your genetics, and your age.

So if you're trying to structure an exercise program, what's the answer? Doing something — anything — is clearly better than doing nothing at all. Aim for at least 30 minutes of activity just about every day. If you're serious about improving your health as much as you possibly can and want to increase your chances of long-term weight loss, aim for an hour of activity daily.

### Question #115: Do I have to work out for 30 consecutive minutes or are shorter workouts just as effective?

*The short answer:* Good news for this time-crunched world we live in: You don't have to do your entire exercise routine all in one shot to lose some weight or reap cardiovascular benefits.

*Extensive evidence* now suggests that accumulating physical activity in short, intermittent bouts can be just as effective as continuous exercise for increasing overall fitness. Consider a University of Wisconsin study that divided 30 overweight college students into three groups. One group did three 10-minute exercise sessions a day, five days a week. The second group did two 15-minute exercise sessions, and the third did one 30-minute session. All of the groups exercised at 75 percent of maximum effort. After eight weeks, all three groups lost the same amount of weight — between 11 and 19.5 pounds — and realized the same gains in cardio fitness.

Clearly, 10-minute bouts of exercise won't turn you into a world-class athlete (but then again, neither will 30-minute bouts). However, if your goal is to fit in the daily half-hour of cardio exercise recommended for general health and fitness, there's no reason you have to do those 30 minutes consecutively. If several mini-workouts fit into your schedule better than one long session, go for it.

### Question #116: Can I get in shape by doing gardening, housework, and other so-called "lifestyle activities"?

*The short answer:* The research is inconclusive. We think every little bit helps, although you can't expect to train for a 10-k by dusting the living room or poking around in the garden.

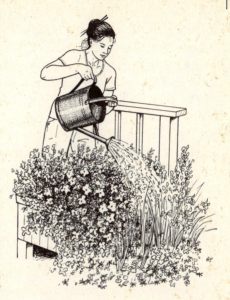

*For nearly three decades* several health authorities, including the U.S. Surgeon General, have advocated "exercise-lite" activities as an alternative to a more vigorous exercise program. Their pitch: Incorporating at least 30 minutes of movement, including gardening and housework, into your life on most days can help prevent disease, control weight, and increase stamina. The Surgeon General is not suggesting that fertilizing your lawn equates to running a marathon but rather that some amount of movement — *any* amount — is preferable to being a Coca-Cola–carrying member of the couch-potato club.

The evidence? In some large, landmark studies, folks who did at least 30 minutes a day of somewhat challenging movement, whether it was brisk walking or pulling weeds, were significantly less likely to die of heart disease than those who did little more than flex their index finger to change channels. People who were super-fit did have the lowest death rates, but all their extra work gained them only a 10 percent to 15 percent advantage over the moderately fit group.

Exercise-lite advocates also point to a study conducted at the Cooper Institute for Aerobic Research. Researchers randomly assigned some 200 sedentary men and woman to one of two groups: the "lifestyle" group, which was encouraged to do things like use the stairs instead of the escalator, and the "structured" group, which did a vigorous gym workout at least three days a week. To the researchers' surprise, the exercise-lite group slimmed down slightly more than the structured group, reducing their body fat by 2.4 percent over 16 weeks, compared with 1.9 percent for the structured group. (Both groups lost about one clothing size.) The liters also lowered their blood pressure a bit more.

The exercise-lite group may have been more successful, the researchers suspect, because it's more convenient to do snippets of activity here and there rather than arrange your whole schedule around a workout. Many people drop out of structured routines because they simply find it too hard to make it a habit.

But before you cancel your gym membership, consider the other side of the story. Some experts believe that exercise lite is to regular exercise what Snackwell cookies are to low-fat eating: a poor substitute for the real thing. They worry that instead of encouraging people to become more active, the exercise-lite message has given people an excuse to do as little as possible.

There is some evidence to suggest that exercise lite is of little use, including a study that followed more than 2,000 women. Although three-quarters of the women met the standards for exercise-lite recommendations, mainly through heavy-duty housework, they were no less likely to be overweight or have a lower resting heart rate (defined in Question #123) than those who did little to no activity at all. Only those who walked briskly for at least 30 minutes a day seemed to benefit from their activity.

At this point, researchers are still sorting this issue out. We think the best-case scenario is to support a regular, structured exercise routine with a foundation of lifestyle activity. And if you're a lounge lizard whose idea of exercise is standing up while you microwave a burrito, then spending some time each day planting, digging, and pulling up weeds can help you get healthier. Who knows? It may also inspire you to transition into a more formal exercise program.

## Question #117: Is it okay to do an aerobic workout every day?

*The short answer:* If your typical workout is a brisk walk or a leisurely bike ride that lasts less than an hour, it's fine to exercise every day. But if longer or more strenuous workouts are part of your workout program, we suggest taking one or two days off a week.

*Unless you're working out* at supersonically high intensity, cardio exercise doesn't usually tear down muscles the same way lifting weights does. However, when you work out in the upper ranges of your target zone (defined in Question #119) too often or for too long, you not only increase your chances of injury, but you also risk mental burnout and compromise your immune system. So here's our rule of thumb: If you do some of your workouts at 75 percent of your maximum heart rate or above or if you do several weekly workouts of any intensity that last longer than an hour, take at least one full day off from exercise a week. Think of rest as an important part of a balanced, sensible workout routine, a sort of yin to your exercise yang, a chance to let your body recover and recharge.

No matter what your workout program or fitness level, always, *always* take a day off when your body tells you to, whether it's scheduled into your PalmPilot or not. This doesn't mean allowing your butt to park itself in front of the TV whenever it so desires. But when your knees are achy or your muscles feel like they belong in a Salvador Dali painting, a little downtime is probably what you need to get back in the swing.

## Question #118: How do I know if I'm pushing myself hard enough when I exercise?

*The short answer:* You can monitor your intensity level in several ways, ranging from the very low-tech "talk test" to using a super-fancy heart-rate monitor.

*Many exercisers,* especially inexperienced ones, don't intuitively know how much effort they're exerting. So they either overdo it to the point of extreme soreness (not to mention developing a hate-hate relationship with exercise), or go at such a sluglike pace that they never see results. Keeping an eye on your workout intensity can help you find that middle ground between "exercise maniac" and "total slacker." It also gives you a sense of your progress. When running a 10-minute mile doesn't wear you out like it used to, that's a sign that your fitness is improving.

The easiest way to get a read on your exercise intensity is to take the "talk test": simply try having a conversation. If you can blabber endlessly, like a teenager on a cell phone, you're slacking off; pick up the pace or your heart and lungs won't even know you've worked out. On the other hand, if you're so winded that you can barely utter "Oxygen!" you need to scale back your effort. Otherwise, you may end up with more aches, pains, and injuries than you bargained for, and you're likely to burn out on this exercise thing fairly quickly.

If you're a low-tech kind of person and don't like fussing with charts or gadgets, the talk test is a reasonable self-check. However, if at some point you want a more precise read on your exercise effort, we recommend monitoring your heart rate — the number of times your heart beats per minute. Your heart rate is a pretty accurate measure of how hard you're exercising; the faster your heart thumps, the more effort your body is exerting to keep you moving. You can measure your heart rate by taking your pulse while you exercise or, better yet, strapping a heart-rate monitor to your chest. (You can also estimate your heart rate with a method called RPE, described in Question #125.)

To take your pulse, lightly press your first two fingers (not your thumb, since it contains a pulse of its own) on the artery that's close to the base of your thumb, and feel the thumping. Most people can see this artery as a bluish line that runs down the outside of the palm side of the wrist just under the skin's surface. Count the number of beats for 15 seconds and multiply this number by 4. You now have your heart rate. Although many group-exercise instructors use a 10- or 6-second count, these methods can magnify any error that results from miscounting beats.

You may see people taking their pulse at their neck instead of their wrist. This method is less accurate because the artery found at the neck has built-in pressure receptors. Pressing your fingers against it signals the receptors to slow your pulse down. That said, even the wrist method is not always so accurate. Some people just can't seem to feel or "hear" the thumping or have trouble keeping track of the beats, since they come so quickly while you're exercising. You may end up counting your footsteps instead of your heartbeats. One solution is to stop exercising so you can better focus on taking your pulse, but this poses a problem, too: If you stop, your pulse begins to slow down, so you're still not getting an accurate reading.

For these reasons, you may want to wear a heart-rate monitor, a gizmo that reads your heart's electrical activity and transmits the information to a receiver that you wear on your wrist. With a quick glance at your wrist, you instantly know exactly how fast your heart is beating. Monitors cost about $50 to $400, depending on how many bells and whistles you want. Some cardio machines are now compatible with Polar heart-rate monitors; you wear the strap around your chest and the signal goes to the display panel, which takes the place of the wrist receiver. Other machines dispense with the need for a chest strap, displaying your heart rate when you place your palms on the handles.

Of course, knowing your heart rate at any given moment is one thing, but what do you do with this information? How do you know what number to aim for? That's where your "target zone" comes in. (See Question #119 for an explanation.)

## Question #119: What exactly is the *target zone*?

*The short answer:* Your target zone, also known as your "target heart-rate zone" and "target training zone," is a range of heart rates you should try to stay within while you're exercising so that you get optimal fitness benefits without risking overexertion or injury. Even within this zone, it's a good idea to vary your intensity.

*Most experts,* including the American College of Sports Medicine, recommend a target zone of 60 percent to 90 percent of your maximum heart rate (a.k.a. your "max," the fastest your heart can possibly beat), although there are exceptions to this rule. For instance, if you are just starting an exercise program, working at 60 percent of your maximum heart rate may be too exhausting. In this case, stay closer to 50 percent or 55 percent of your max until you're more fit. Some heart-rate monitors come with an alarm that can be set to beep when you exceed or fall below the target zone that you set.

There are some instances when you might want to exercise at above 90 percent of your max, perhaps as high as 95 percent. For instance, when you do intervals (defined in Question #129), train for an athletic event, or aim to get to the next level of fitness, you might want to throw in short spurts of very high intensity exercise, lasting from 30 seconds to 5 minutes. Use these near-max efforts sparingly, however. The closer you get to your max in a workout, the more likely you are to blow out a knee or sustain some other sort of injury due to the higher demands placed on your body.

Many serious athletes break their target zones into a series of mini-zones — for instance, 60 to 70 percent of max, 70 to 80 percent of max, 80 to 90 percent of max, and above 90 percent. They follow training programs that dictate how much time they spend in each zone during various phases of their training. To find out more about determining your mini-zones, check out Web sites such as heartzones.com and trainingbible.com.

## Question #120: What's the easiest way to calculate my target zone?

*The short answer:* The simplest, though not the most accurate, way is to estimate your maximum heart rate by subtracting your age from 220, then calculating 60 percent and 90 percent of this number. However, this method, the "age-predicted" formula, can be quite inaccurate for many people, so compare your results with the other methods described in this chapter.

*Here's how a 40-year-old* would do the calculations using the "age-predicted" formula:

$$220 - 40 = 180, \text{estimated maximum heart rate}$$
$$180 \times .60 = 108, \text{low end of target zone}$$
$$180 \times .90 = 162, \text{high end of target zone}$$

So if you're 40, according to this formula your heart rate should stay between 108 and 162 beats per minute most of the time you're exercising.

Consider the numbers a very rough estimate. Your true "max" might be as much as 15 beats higher or lower. In other words, if you're 40, your max may actually be as high as 195 or as low as 165, which means that the target zone you calculate using this formula may be way off base, and you may end up overestimating or underestimating how hard you are truly working. This formula has remained popular over the years because it's simple, but it was developed based on studies that included smokers and people with heart disease and was never intended to be used by the public to gauge appropriate intensity levels for exercising. Another problem with this formula is that it assumes that your max will decrease by about one beat per year, which isn't true for everyone.

Also, this formula tends to be most accurate for activities in which your feet hit the ground. When you ride a bike, your maximum heart rate is about 5 beats slower than when you run. This is because cycling uses fewer muscle groups than running, so your muscles pump blood through your body a bit more slowly and with less force. Most people have different maximums for different activities. When you swim, your max might be 10 or more beats slower than when you run. Scientists aren't completely clear on why this is, but the going theory is that water creates additional pressure on the body and its blood vessels, so your heart pumps a bit more slowly to circulate blood throughout your body.

In other words, the heart may be working just as hard as it would on land, but it may register 10 beats lower for the same amount of effort.

## Question #121: What is the most accurate way to find my target zone?

*The short answer:* The most accurate way is to base your target zone on a "maximum stress test" conducted by a physician or a trained fitness professional under the supervision of a physician. However, all of the methods described below are more accurate than the formula described in the previous question.

*With a maximum stress test,* you run on a treadmill while your heart rate is measured as the speed and/or incline of the machine is gradually increased. Either you wear a heart-rate monitor or you're strapped to a machine with a slew of electrodes. The point at which your heart rate stops increasing, even when the speed or incline increases, is the fastest your heart is capable of beating and is therefore your true maximum heart rate. At best, this test is extremely uncomfortable. At worst, you feel like your organs are about to spontaneously combust.

How long this test takes depends on your max. If you're not very fit, you're going to max out at a lower speed/grade combination and you'll be done in a few minutes. If you're in great shape, it's going to take you longer. There are some Olympic athletes who have outlasted some of the tests; in other words, the program designed to measure their max went as high as it could but the athlete could still keep up! Some tests, however, are humanly impossible to beat. Different testing facilities use different protocols.

Could you do this sort of test on your own, without going to the trouble of making a doctor's appointment? Yes, although we strongly recommend against doing this unless you've been exercising for a good while and have clearance from your doctor. To conduct your own all-out test, you'll need a heart-rate monitor and a pretty high pain threshold. It's a lot harder to force yourself to go full speed ahead on your own than it is to keep up with an intensity level that someone else has set. If you have trouble pushing your limits outside of competitive situations or being chased by a swarm of killer bees, you'll have trouble determining your max on your own.

After you warm up, gradually increase your intensity until you reach the point where you are pushing as hard as you possibly can. The highest heart rate you achieve within about 20 minutes is probably pretty close to your maximum heart rate. There are several books that offer detailed instruction on how to do a self-test to find your heart rate for various activities, including running, biking, and swimming.

If you aren't keen on the idea of pushing to the point of suffering but still want a somewhat accurate estimate of your maximum heart rate, you may be a candidate for a "submax test," conducted by a trainer at a gym. With this test, usually done on a bike or treadmill, you exercise from 3 to 20 minutes (depending on your fitness and the type of test being performed), gradually increasing your intensity. Once your heart rate reaches a certain below-maximum level, your tester will use a series of formulas to extrapolate what your maximum would be. A submax test isn't as accurate as a max test, but it's significantly more accurate than simply using a mathematical formula. You can also do a variety of submax tests on yourself and then average the result to increase accuracy. A number of these tests are described at heartzones.com.

And finally, speaking of formulas, there is one considered more accurate than the age-predicted method described above. It's called the Karvonen formula and is considered superior because it factors in your resting heart rate, which is a rough estimate of fitness. As you become more fit, your resting heart rate generally drops and you are capable of exercising at a greater intensity. Top endurance athletes have resting heart rates as low as 30 beats per minute (bpm), whereas a sedentary person may have a resting heart rate of 80 bpm. In other words, a couch potato's heart may have to work more than twice as hard to pump the same amount of blood as an elite athlete's. Keep in mind that your heart rate is in large part genetically determined. If your resting heart rate is 60 and your friend's is 52, this doesn't necessarily mean that your friend is in better shape. Instead of comparing your resting heart rate to someone else's, compare it to your own resting heart rate as you become more fit.

By using a formula that factors in your resting heart rate, you will end up with a target zone that is a more accurate reflection of your true training zone. We recommend recalculating with the Karvonen formula every six months or so, to see if you need to tweak your target heart-rate zone.

Here's how to calculate your target zone using the Karvonen method.

1. Take your pulse at rest for one full minute, either when you wake up in the morning or after you've been sitting quietly for several minutes. (See Question #118 for instructions on taking your pulse.) Or, use a heart-rate monitor. Let's say your resting heart rate is 60 beats per minute.

2. Figure out your age-predicted maximum by subtracting your age from 220. If you're 40, your age-predicted max is 180.

3. Subtract your resting heart rate from your age-predicted maximum: 180 − 60 = 120

4. Multiply the answer you got in step 3 by .60 and .90. Following our example, you get 72 and 108.

5. Add your resting heart rate back to both answers you got in step 4. This is your estimated target zone:

   $$72 + 60 = 132, \text{low end}$$
   $$108 + 60 = 168, \text{high end}$$

Compared with the standard age-predicted formula, the Karvonen method calculates higher target heart rates for people with higher resting heart rates. At first this seems like a paradox; why should less fit people be working out at a greater intensity than more fit exercisers? But actually, that's not the case.

The higher your resting heart rate, the narrower the gap between your resting heart rate and the low end of your Karvonen-predicted training range. For instance, the low end of the zone for a 40-year-old with a resting heart of 60 is 132 bpm, whereas for a 40-year-old with a resting heart rate of 90, the low end is 144. So, even though the training range is higher for the person with the 90 bpm heart rate, this less fit person enters his or her training range more quickly.

The entire training range for a less fit person is also narrower than for a fitter person. Our 40-year-old with a resting heart rate of 60 has a Karvonen-calculated target zone that spans 36 beats, whereas our 40-year-old with a resting heart rate of 90 has a range that spans a mere 27 beats.

# Question #122: What is the *fat-burning zone*?

*The short answer:* It's a misleading concept based on the erroneous assumption that you'll burn more fat if you exercise at a slower pace.

*Hanging on the walls* of some health clubs and appearing on some treadmills and other cardio machine displays you'll find a chart that divides your target zone into two sub-zones: the "fat-burning zone" (the lower half of your target zone) and the "cardio zone" (the upper half). The suggestion is that low-intensity exercise burns more fat than high-intensity exercise. This is not true. To find out why, flip to Question #53.

# Question #123: Is it true that the lower my resting heart rate, the better shape I'm in?

*The short answer:* Sort of. Your resting heart rate will decrease as your fitness level improves. However, resting heart rate has a strong genetic component, so you can't judge a person's fitness solely by the number of times per minute his or her heart beats.

*Most people's resting heart rates* fall between 60 and 90 beats per minute. Although many fit people do have resting heart rates in the range of 40 to 50 beats per minute or even lower, it's not uncommon for even world-class athletes to have much higher resting heart rates.

Regardless of what your resting heart rate is when you start exercising, you can expect it to decrease after several months of training. The amount it drops depends on your starting point (the higher your resting heart rate, the more room it has to drop) as well as your training program. If your pulse is 80 beats per minute before you begin a regular workout routine, you might expect a 5- to 10-beat decrease after several months of training. Your cardiovascular system becomes more efficient, so your heart needs fewer pumps per minute to circulate your blood.

Resting heart rate is very sensitive to medication, lack of sleep, stress, and caffeine. Taking certain thyroid medications, for instance, can elevate your resting heart rate by as much as 40 beats per minute. For the most accurate measure, take your resting heart rate when you first wake up, before eating or drinking anything, especially caffeinated beverages. If it's consistently over 120 bpm, check in with your doctor.

## Question #124: How long should it take my heart rate to return to normal after a workout?

*The short answer:* The time will vary, but in general, the faster your heart rate slows down after exercise, the better shape your cardiovascular system is in.

*Your recovery heart rate* is a good way to gauge your fitness level; in fact, it's a better gauge than your resting heart rate. The heart rate of a fit person will begin to slow down almost immediately after finishing an exercise session, whereas the heart rate of an unfit exerciser may take hours to return to normal.

One way to measure your progress is to track your recovery heart rate. This is easiest to do if you're wearing a heart-rate monitor, but you can also use the manual method described in Question #118. Glance at your heart rate immediately after the workout and then again 1 minute later. Chart your numbers for a month or so, and if you're working out regularly, you should see the difference between the two heart rates gradually increase. In the beginning, your heart rate may drop only 10 beats in the first minute, but after a month or so, you might see a 20- or 30-beat decrease.

Keep in mind that this is a good gauge only if you're comparing similar workouts. If you exercise harder or longer than usual, it may take longer for your heart rate to return to normal.

## Question #125: I find it a hassle to check my heart rate when I work out. Is there a simpler way for me to gauge how hard I'm working?

*The short answer:* Try RPE, short for "relative perceived exertion" or "rating of perceived exertion." It's a low-tech method of gauging exercise intensity and is a good substitute for taking your pulse.

*If you don't want to bother* with a heart-rate monitor or periodic pulse check, try rating your workout effort on the RPE scale of 1 to 10 — 1 being very easy, like sitting on the couch watching *The Princess Bride,* and 10 being so maxed out that you feel you can't continue moving for more than a few seconds. Most of your workouts should rate between a 5 and an 8, a range that, with some practice, should correlate well with your target zone (defined in Question #119). Studies show that when people assign a 4 rating to their workout, they are typically exercising at about 60 to 65 percent of their maximum heart rate. A 7 or 8 rating corresponds closely with a heart rate that's 85 to 90 percent of max.

Beginners should aim for the low end of the 4-to-8 range. If you're relatively fit, vary your workouts so that you spend about 20 percent of your workout time in the upper reaches of your zone. You can do this either by spending 20 percent of each work-

## Rating of Perceived Exertion (RPE)

| Level | Heart Rate | RPE | Talk Test |
| --- | --- | --- | --- |
| Easy | 50–60% | 2–3 | Talking (even singing) is easy. |
| Moderate | 60–70% | 4–5 | You are still able to talk but it takes a little more effort. |
| Challenging | 70–80% | 6–7 | Breathing is challenged and you are not inclined to chat. |
| Very challenging | 80–90% | 8–9 | You are panting pretty hard and conversation is nearly impossible. |
| Near maximum to maximum | 90% and above | 10 | You can't sustain this intensity for more than a few seconds. |

out at a higher intensity or by doing one workout a week at the high end of the range (after a low-intensity warm-up, of course). If you're in top shape or gearing up for a big event, you might do two or three workouts a week where you spend time working in the upper zones. (However, you don't want to do this year round because it can lead to injury and burnout.) To start, it's helpful to have an actual 1-to-10 scale posted on the wall, as many gyms do. See the example above. However, you can also mentally picture the scale in your head. After a little practice, that's just as effective.

When you rate your workout effort, be sure to consider the whole picture: how tired your muscles feel, how much you're sweating, how heavily you're breathing, how much you can feel your heart thumping in your chest. Focusing on one aspect alone can be deceiving. Some people breathe heavily when they're not working all that hard, while others don't sweat that much even when they're going like gangbusters.

**Q**uestion #126: I know lactic acid is what gives you "the burn" when you work out. But what exactly is it?

*The short answer:* Lactic acid, or lactate, is a substance that's produced in your cells when your body makes and uses energy.

*Actually, lactic acid* is produced all the time, but you notice it only after an intense weight-training set or an all-out sprint, when it floods into your muscles faster than your bloodstream can carry it out. You can tell when this is happening because lactic acid *is* an acid: When there's a lot of it, you experience a burning, searing pain, as if someone just replaced your blood with boiling coffee. This is your body's way of demanding that you slow down or stop so that your muscles can get back into balance again.

As we explain in Question #198, lactic acid is probably not responsible for the delayed muscle soreness you feel a day or two after a hard workout. Even if you've had a large enough lactic acid pileup to cause your legs to buckle, most of it is cleared out via blood circulation within 15 minutes.

**Q**uestion #127: I've heard coaches and trainers use the terms *anaerobic threshold* and *lactate threshold*. What do these words mean?

*The short answer:* Your lactate threshold is the point during a high-intensity workout when lactic acid begins to enter your bloodstream in quantities above steady-state levels. Your anaerobic threshold is the point at which lactate begins flooding into your bloodstream in major amounts; you begin to use up more oxygen than you can inhale through your lungs (a.k.a. "oxygen debt"), and you begin to produce lactic acid more quickly than you can clear it from your muscles.

*When you're exercising* at your lactate threshold you know it: Your heart begins to beat a lot harder, you begin breathing very deeply, and your muscles start to feel heavy. When you're exercising at your anaerobic threshold you *really* know it: Your heart rate is nearly maxed out, your breathing is ragged, and your muscles feel like cement. If you continue exercising at this level, eventually you have to bail. (Beginners may have to stop right away, whereas more fit people may last 20 minutes or more exercising at their anaerobic threshold.)

Why on earth would anyone want to put up with the discomfort of training at his or her lactate or anaerobic threshold? Because you can build up a tolerance to high-intensity exercise over time, much as you can develop a tolerance for your spouse leaving his or her clothes on the floor. After a while, you start to go anaerobic at higher workout intensities. In other words, you're able to push harder and longer before fatiguing.

You can find out your precise anaerobic and lactate thresholds by getting tested at a lab or specialized training center. The tests aren't cheap — about $200 — and may take 20 minutes to an hour, depending on your fitness level. As you pedal on a bike or run on a treadmill, the tester will gradually increase the intensity of your workout while pricking your finger and extracting blood about every three minutes.

There's no need to go to all this trouble if you're just trying to lose some weight or achieve general fitness goals. But if you're serious about competing, your results can help you or your coach tailor a training program to your fitness level and goals. Your lactate threshold and anaerobic threshold correlate to certain heart-rate levels, so by wearing a heart-rate monitor, you can gauge how hard you're pushing in relation to these intensity markers. Lactate threshold typically occurs at about 80 to 90 percent of maximum heart rate; anaerobic threshold generally occurs at about 95 to 100 percent of maximum heart rate.

**Q**uestion #128: People in the gym talk about their VO2 max, and I've read this term in fitness magazines. What does it mean?

*The short answer:* In tech-speak, VO2 max refers to the maximum volume of oxygen your muscles are capable of processing. In layman's terms, it means your maximum aerobic-exercise intensity — basically the point at which you're sucking wind pretty badly.

*Your VO2 max* is the limit of your ability to perform aerobic exercise — the point right around your anaerobic threshold, a not-so-fun phenomenon we cover in Question #127. It's measured in terms of how much oxygen your body can convert to fuel each minute without having to tap into the anaerobic energy that's stored in your muscles. The way VO2 max is typically expressed — in millimeters of oxygen per kilogram of body weight per minute — won't mean much to the average exerciser, but the numbers are a tool researchers can use to measure things like how much work it takes to pedal a bike compared with running on a treadmill.

Your VO2 max depends on several factors, including your fitness level, genetics, gender, age, and the type of activity you're doing. The more fit you are, the more efficient your body becomes at processing oxygen, and the higher your VO2 max. Someone who walks on the treadmill at a brisk pace five days a week will have a higher VO2 max than someone whose longest walk is from the TV to the refrigerator. The typical unfit person might reach VO2 max running at 6 mph (a 10-minute-mile pace), whereas an elite runner might not reach VO2 max until a speed of 12.5 mph (a 4:48-minute-mile pace) or even faster.

However, your potential for improving your VO2 max comes down to genetics. Most of us wouldn't be able to come anywhere close to the VO2 max levels of Olympians even if we spent years training alongside these genetically gifted athletes.

Women tend to have VO2 max levels 15 to 20 percent lower than men, primarily because they have smaller hearts, less blood volume, and less muscle mass to saturate with oxygen. As you get older you experience a drop in VO2 max by about 9 percent per decade after the age of 20, although it's not clear whether this drop is related to the aging process or the fact that as you get older, you tend to spend more time sitting on your butt than bouncing up and down in a mosh pit. You also have higher VO2 measurements for some activities than for others. Unless you're a trained cyclist, your VO2 max will probably be higher for running than for pedaling on a bike because running uses more of your muscles at one time.

Is there any reason for the average exerciser to find out his or her VO2 max? Well, it's one more way to gauge your fitness level. If you're curious about your VO2, you may be able to get it tested by a physician or by an exercise scientist in a lab at the same time you get tested for your maximum heart rate. Some tests measure maximum heart rate and VO2 max simultaneously by hooking you up to a machine that compares the amount of oxygen in the air you inhale and the amount of oxygen in the air you exhale. Since the difference is how much oxygen you were able to use up, it's an excellent measure of VO2.

Even if you don't go through this very uncomfortable process, which involves having a plastic tube shoved in your mouth and a plastic clip clamped onto the bridge of your nose, a knowledgeable fitness trainer can help you estimate your VO2 max, since it has a strong correlation with your true maximum heart rate. (Finding your VO2 max with this method involves some complicated math and isn't as on-the-money as a direct measurement.) Incidentally, VO2 also has a linear relationship with how many calories you're burning. In fact, researchers measure VO2 and translate the figures into accurate calorie-burn estimations.

**Question #129: Is it true that interval training can help boost your calorie burn? What is this type of training, and how do I go about doing it?**

*The short answer:* Interval training is fitness-speak for mixing spurts of high-intensity exercise with periods of lower-intensity exercise.

*Although running at high speed* for 20 minutes burns a lot of calories, most exercisers can't sustain a killer pace for that long. On the other hand, lollygagging through the mall for 20 minutes won't overtax most of us, but it's hardly going to incinerate calories. Interval training gives you the best of both worlds: You boost your calorie burn — and your fitness level — without flaming out. Since your body recovers between efforts, you can last a lot longer without feeling winded or risking injury. Recovering with low-intensity exercise is generally better than stopping altogether because it helps your muscles flush out waste products, like lactic acid, that are built up during high-intensity work. Interval training is key for progressing in running, cycling, swimming, and other aerobic endeavors. Without it, you'll have a harder time moving up to the next level of fitness.

If you're new to interval training, try a 1:3 sprint:rest pattern. On the treadmill, for instance, run for 1 minute at a speedy pace, then jog or walk for 3 minutes at an easy pace. Repeat the cycle three to five times, gradually increasing the number of interval cycles as you become more fit. Another way to make intervals tougher is to take less rest in between. For instance, as you get in better shape, you might sprint for 3 minutes and jog for 2 minutes. Always do a thorough warm-up before you start your intervals.

There are countless ways to structure an interval workout, depending on your goals, time constraints, and fitness level. Just don't do more than one or two interval workouts a week. Your body needs time to reboot between workouts.

## Question #130: Should bottom-heavy women avoid stairclimbers and step aerobics?

*The short answer:* No! Stairclimbing and step aerobics are excellent ways to get fit and burn calories no matter what your body shape.

*Having a large derrière* has more to do with your genetics, your eating habits, and how much (or little) you exercise than with the type of aerobic exercise you do. Both stairclimbing and step aerobics have the potential to burn a lot of calories, which will help reduce — not expand — the size of your bottom. It's true that stairclimbers and step classes work the butt and thighs, but cardiovascular exercise of any type doesn't build much muscle, unless you work against heavy resistance and have a predisposition to developing large muscles in the first place.

Sure, if you pile a huge stack of risers underneath your step or take slow, deep steps on the stairclimber as if you're slogging through a waist-high snowdrift, you might build up your butt — the same way you'll build up your quads on a bike if you pedal slowly against heavy resistance. But a typical fast-paced step or stairclimbing workout isn't going to do anything but help burn off the fat covering those glutes or any other part of your body. And if you do happen to have an extreme genetic tendency to develop muscle, well, personally we feel there are worse problems to be faced with than a shapely butt and a muscular pair of thighs.

## Question #131: Why do my toes sometimes tingle or feel numb when I exercise on cardio machines?

*The short answer:* You may be compressing nerves in your feet.

*Toe numbness seems to be fairly common,* especially among the stairclimbing set. In a survey of 212 frequent stairclimbing machine users, Stanford University researchers found that 39 percent of the exercisers reported experiencing some level of forefoot numbness while stairclimbing. The condition typically disappeared, either as the exercisers continued to climb or when the exercise session ended. The researchers concluded that the condition, known as transient paresthesia, was probably caused by compression of the nerves located between the toes, due to persistent and prolonged weight bearing on the forefoot. Because your foot position is similar on the elliptical machine, you may encounter similar problems on this machine, too. Stairclimber and elliptical manufacturers have tried to remedy the problem by making foot plates softer, flatter, and wider.

Numbness is annoying but typically isn't dangerous. In fact, you can probably alleviate or even eliminate the symptoms by maintaining a flat-footed position, as opposed to keeping your heel lifted off the pedals, and by wearing shoes that provide ample width at the toe. Some people find relief by wearing light, flexible running shoes that allow your toes some wiggle room and don't hold your arch too firmly in place, while others find shoes with extra shock absorption a big help. Some companies have begun making athletic shoes with an extra-flexible forefoot to address the numbness problem. Thin socks that don't fit too snugly may also do the trick; so may loosening your shoelaces.

If wiggling your toes doesn't get rid of the numbness, try getting off the machine for a moment and walking around a bit to get the blood flowing into your toes. Once the tingling subsides, continue exercising.

## Question #132: As I become more fit, will I sweat more — or less — than I used to?

*The short answer:* Whether you're drenched in sweat or barely glowing depends more on your genetics than on your fitness level, although the fitter you become, the more you're likely to perspire during exercise.

*Some people are so sweaty* after a 4-mile jog on the treadmill that they look like they got caught in a torrential downpour. Others can finish the same workout looking so fresh they could probably head straight to the office without even showering. (No comment about how they might smell.) The difference is primarily due to how active a person's sweat glands are, which is genetically determined.

Still, your fitness level can influence how much you sweat. In general, the fitter you are, the earlier in the workout and the more profusely you're likely to perspire. Sweating is your body's cooling system. A fit person's body will recognize the buildup of heat sooner and work up a sweat to avoid overheating. Fit people also tend to sweat more because they're capable of working at higher intensity levels, which, in turn, generates more heat and requires more sweating.

How much you sweat also is influenced by the weather conditions. On hot, humid days, you're likely to sweat buckets, especially when there's no wind. The more you sweat during exercise — whether it's due to active sweat glands, a high fitness level, or Florida-in-July conditions — the more fluids you need to guzzle before, during, and after your workout.

Finally, don't confuse sweating with fat burning. Some people wear plastic suits or sweatshirts when they work out because they believe that excess sweating will help them lose weight. This isn't true. When you sweat, you lose water weight, not fat, and you'll regain the pounds as soon as you replenish your fluids. What's more, wearing heavy clothing, especially when it's rubberized or plastic, can be dangerous, potentially leading to serious dehydration or even heat stroke.

## Question #133: I never saw an elliptical machine until a few years ago, and now they seem really popular. Where did they come from?

*The short answer:* The first elliptical was designed by an engineer in an effort to rehab his track-star daughter's knee injury.

*In the weird-history department,* the elliptical trainer can't beat the stairclimber, which was developed in the late 1800s as a way of generating power for prisons and as a form of punishment for inmates. Still, the elliptical machine has an intriguing story behind it.

The elliptical's unique, oval-shaped stride was invented in the early 1990s by an engineer whose daughter injured her knee while running high-school track. In an effort to understand her biomechanics, he filmed her running on a treadmill. When he plotted a graph of the range of motion her feet went through during each stride, he noticed it was shaped like an ellipse. Armed with this information, he built the first elliptical training machine, a crude contraption with a choppy, limited stride and wood planks for foot plates.

Ultimately, the engineer's elliptical trainer prototype found its way into the research and development "think tank" at Precor, a large exercise equipment manufacturer best known for making high-quality stationary bikes and treadmills. Although the design was rough, it sparked excitement in the Precor engineers.

The engineers spent three years transforming the first elliptical designs into a viable exercise machine. They consulted with exercise physiologists, gym owners, and everyday exercisers, incorporating their feedback to refine the stride length, foot plate size, and every other aspect of the machine's design. During this process, they added an incline feature to vary muscle usage.

In 1995, Precor unveiled its first commercial elliptical model at a trade show in Chicago, and within 15 minutes, there were lines out the door of people waiting to try it. The exercising public liked the no-impact gliding motion of the Precor elliptical trainer right away, and the machine quickly overtook the stationary cycle and stairclimber, becoming the second-most-popular piece of equipment (behind the treadmill) in the gym. Today, more than two dozen companies sell elliptical trainers for both the gym and home use, although Precor machines are still by far the most popular.

## Question #134: Is there any advantage to exercising backward?

*The short answer:* No.

*Backward exercising* — a.k.a. "retro" exercising — has always attracted a small but enthusiastic following. There's an annual backward mile run in Central Park on April Fools' Day and an entire Web site devoted to backward running (backward-running-backward.com). And some years back, a group of die-hards even proposed to the International Olympic Committee that a backward marathon be introduced into the Olympic Games. Lately exercising in reverse has become all the rage indoors because of elliptical trainers and Spinning bikes that allow you to pedal both backward and forward.

What's with all this reverse physiology? Rumor has it that exercising backward works your butt and hamstrings (rear thigh muscles) more effectively than pedaling forward. Turns out, the rumor is false. Computer analysis shows that it's actually the quadriceps (front thigh muscles) that do most of the work during backward exercising, while the glutes and hamstrings are virtually taken out of the equation. A University of Oregon study on the elliptical trainer found that pedaling forward works the glutes a whopping 33 percent more than pedaling backward. A much better way to tone your glutes would be to walk straight ahead to the weight room and do some strengthening exercises such as squats and lunges.

Retro exercise also increases your risk for injury. Pedaling backward on the elliptical machine puts extra pressure on your knees and is not recommended by Precor, the company that invented the machine. Some of the knockoff brands tout the "dual direction forward and backward elliptical action," but a Precor representative told us that the option to stride backward was just a byproduct of the belt-drive mechanism rather than an intentionally engineered feature.

Backpedaling on a Spinning bike is also a backward idea. The toe clips are designed to keep your feet firmly anchored in the pedals, but they work only when you pedal forward. Spinning backward increases the chances that your feet will disengage and the pedal cranks will whack you in the shins. The manufacturers of Spinning bikes became so alarmed by the number of bruised and bloodied ankles caused in this manner that they launched a campaign warning instructors to cease the practice.

As for backward running, competing in the Central Park Backward Mile race may be a fun change of pace, but don't make this form of exercise a habit. Since you don't have eyes in back of your head, you tend to run with your body slightly twisted so you can see where you're going. This awkward motion throws your posture out of whack, potentially wreaking havoc on your lower back. You can't keep it up for long periods of time without feeling tired, frustrated, and, in some cases, dizzy.

If you really want to exercise backward, do it the old-fashioned way: Get in the pool and swim the backstroke.

# Question #135: Which delivers a better workout, an upright stationary cycle or a recumbent stationary cycle?

*The short answer:* Both types of bikes can whip you into cardio-vascular shape, although they emphasize different muscle groups. You probably burn more calories per minute on an upright model.

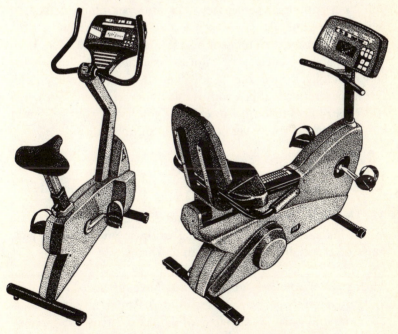

*An upright bike (left) places emphasis on the thigh muscles.*
*A recumbent bike (right) emphasizes the buttocks muscles.*

*On an upright bike,* your thighs and calves do most of the work, but when you pedal a recumbent — a bike with a bucket set and the pedals out in front — your butt muscles get more into the act.

A 150-pound person typically burns between 5 and 9 calories per minute during a moderate-intensity workout on an upright bike, compared with 4 to 7 calories per minute on a recumbent. The slightly reclined position of the recumbent makes it more difficult to get your heart rate elevated; the lower heart rate for the same amount of effort translates into fewer calories burned. The bucket seat provides more support, so you don't expend as much energy keeping your body stable.

Beware of the calorie readouts on recumbent bikes. Since there's been very little research done on this piece of equipment, many manufacturers seem to use the well-established calorie-burn formulas for the upright bike. The limited amount of study that has been done on the stationary recumbent cycle indicates that you'll burn about 20 percent fewer calories per minute compared with an upright cycle.

Consider using a recumbent bike if you have a bad back. Even though you may burn fewer calories per minute, you'll probably stay on it longer since your back will be cushioned and supported. But not everyone will be comfortable on a recumbent. Since you bend your knees toward your chest as you pedal, your belly may get in the way if you're very overweight or pregnant.

## Question #136: Is inline skating a good fitness activity?

*The short answer:* Yes. Skating at a moderate intensity does a fine job of increasing stamina, burning calories, and working your muscles, especially the inner and outer thighs.

*Most studies involving inline skating* have measured how often and how severely participants get injured. Apparently researchers are more interested in the pileup of damaged wrists, fractured elbows, and scraped knees than they are in knowing how skating stacks up as a fitness activity. The few studies that have been done show that inline skating can indeed whip you into shape, provided your skating workout gets your heart beating within its target zone.

A University of Wisconsin Medical School study compared the effects of jogging, cycling, and skating by having 11 volunteers participate in each activity for 30 minutes at heart rates around 150. Researchers concluded that inline skating delivered a more effective aerobic workout than cycling, since the cyclists tended to coast more than the skaters. Likewise, running worked the heart and lungs better than skating, since the skaters glided at times whereas the runners exercised continuously. However, skaters (like cyclists) can increase the aerobic results of their outings by gliding less and skating harder or on uphill terrain.

Other studies show inline skating builds and tones hip and thigh muscles — especially the hamstrings, inner thighs, and outer thighs — in a way that running and cycling do not. When skaters incorporate a strong arm swing, they also get an upper arm and shoulder workout. As for calorie burn, the Wisconsin study found that inline skating at a steady pace burns about 570 calories an hour, even more when you incorporate interval training (defined in Question #129).

## Question #137: How did the marathon distance come to be 26.2 miles?

*The short answer:* It's a long story involving ancient Greek warriors and a high-maintenance British princess.

*Marathon is a coastal village* in Greece about 25 miles from Athens. Back in 490 B.C., after Greek fighters in Marathon conquered a fleet of invading Persians, a messenger named Pheidippides was sent to Athens to report the victory to the king. After running the distance and announcing, "We have won!" he promptly dropped dead.

Fast-forward to 1896, the year of the first modern Olympic Games, held in Athens. To commemorate Pheidippides' historic journey, a running race was held on the unpaved 25-mile road from Marathon to the Olympic stadium in downtown Athens. The "marathon" distance remained 25 miles for the next two Olympic Games. In 1908, when the games were held in London, the course was designed so that the royal family could witness the start of the race on the grounds of Windsor Castle. The Princess of Wales insisted that the runners start directly beneath the castle's nursery windows so that her children could watch the festivities. In order for the runners to finish at the Olympic stadium, the course had to be extended to 26 miles and 385 yards. The distance stuck.

Incidentally, an American from Boston participated in the 1896 Olympic marathon and decided to organize a marathon in his hometown the following year. The Boston Marathon was born and is today the oldest continuously held marathon.

Question #138: Sometimes I hear runners talking about their speed; other times they talk about their pace. What's the difference?

*The short answer:* Speed refers to how much ground you're able to cover in an hour. Pace refers to how fast you complete 1 mile or kilometer.

*Speed is usually measured* in miles per hour or kilometers per hour. So if you walk for an hour and cover 3.5 miles, your walking speed is 3.5 miles per hour. Pace is typically measured in minutes per mile or kilometers per mile. If it takes you 17 minutes to walk one mile, you're walking at a 17-minute-per-mile pace.

Both of these measurements are usually represented on a treadmill display. In the world of running and racing, pace is more important than speed. You might hear someone referred to with admiration as a 6-minute miler; that means she runs a mile in 6 minutes. To convert pace to speed, simply divide 60 (as in 60 minutes in one hour) by your pace. To convert speed to pace, divide 60 by your speed.

## Question #139: What causes "side stitches" during exercise, and how can I get rid of them?

*The short answer:* The reasons for side stitches run the gamut: gas, gulping water too quickly, drinking fluids high in carbohydrate, lack of electrolytes, exercising at too high an intensity, and diaphragm muscle tightness. Whatever the cause, slowing down or pinching the offending area while exhaling forcefully often cures the problem.

*You probably know the feeling:* You're jogging along and feeling fine when suddenly — bam! — it's as if someone started whacking you on the side with a log. What's going on? These piercing cramps, a.k.a. side stitches, usually happen when the ligaments of the muscles that force food through your digestive tract seize up. Side stitches aren't well understood, and it's not clear why some people seem to be more prone to them than others. They often hit exercisers in hot, humid weather and frequently right after they've taken a large slug of water or other fluid. Other people get them when they exercise at a higher intensity than usual or if they're toward the end of a long workout, like at the 24th mile of a marathon.

You can try to avoid stitches by taking small, frequent sips of water or a sports drink while you exercise. Your tummy is less likely to complain if you give it something familiar to drink, so during a long or hard workout be sure to avoid liquids you haven't tried before, especially if you're sensitive to cramps.

Some sports nutritionists recommend eating a banana the night before or the morning of a long exercise session or race to ensure that your body has plenty of potassium. There's speculation that when you sweat a lot, you can throw off your balance of electrolytes, primarily potassium, and this may lead to a scenario where you find yourself doubled over in pain at the side of the road.

If you do find yourself in the throes of a side stitch, slow down or stop until the pain subsides. You can also try this old runner's trick: As you're moving along, grab the offending area and squeeze it as hard as you can while leaning slightly forward, and exhale forcefully five or six times. Believe it or not, this works a lot of the time. In fact, one study found this method to be nearly 100 percent effective with a group of ten male runners who induced cramps by gulping down large amounts of fluids. It seems that squeezing the abdominal muscles may shut off sensation to the cramped areas.

## Question #140: How can I stay in shape when I'm traveling if there's no equipment around?

*The short answer:* You can pack a few small, light items such as a jump rope and an exercise tube, or you can climb hotel steps and do strength exercises with hotel-room furniture.

*Although most hotels* these days offer some type of exercise equipment, some take great liberties with the term "fitness center." You might end up with a creaky weight contraption and busted treadmill — or a facility that is perpetually "closed for repair." For these occasions it helps to come prepared with your own handy gizmos and a repertoire of moves requiring no equipment. (You can also find a local gym via Web sites such as healthclubs.com, nutricise.com, ymca.net, and 24hourfitness.com.)

On the cardio front, going for a walk or a jog is the obvious solution, but sometimes it's too dark or unsafe or the weather isn't cooperating, in which case your best bet is a jump rope (quality brands include Lifeline and Speedrope). For an investment of $5 to $20, you're guaranteed a killer cardio workout. Just remember to clear enough space in your hotel room so you don't whack that bedside lamp. Before your trip, give yourself a few weeks to practice the footwork and build up rope-jumping tolerance in small increments.

If you're traveling sans jump rope, make use of your hotel stairs. You can walk up a few flights, then walk down to recover.

Or, if you're walking up, say, 10 to 15 flights, take the elevator down to catch your breath, then walk up again, and so on.

Bring plenty of water, since there's little ventilation in a stairwell. For an even tougher workout, run up the steps, wear a light backpack while you walk, or take some flights two steps at a time. (Just don't rely on the handrails to propel yourself up.) One caveat: Even if you've mastered the StairMaster at home, climbing actual steps can leave you incredibly sore. You don't want to hobble into that business meeting you flew all the way across the country to attend.

To maintain your strength on the road, rubber exercise tubes are ideal. For a few extra bucks, you can buy a door attachment to mimic the cable pulley exercises you do at the gym. Two great buys are the Fit for Travel Kit (spriproducts.com) and the Lifeline Tote Gym (bodytrends.com). Both cost about $30 and include accessories and a travel case.

If you don't have a tube, perform exercises using your body weight and gravity as resistance. To work your chest, shoulders, and triceps, do a few sets of pushups. You can work your abs and lower back with a variety of exercises we describe in Question #166 and Question #195. For your legs and butt, try squats and lunges (wear a backpack for added resistance), or do "walking" lunges down the hallway. Just make sure you don't lunge right into any room-service carts. To target your biceps and upper back, you can do biceps curls and one-arm rows with a backpack or bag filled with your blow dryer and John Grisham novels.

Keep in mind, too, that yoga requires no equipment and can be just the antidote for airport stresses, sightseeing overdoses, or power schmoozing with clients.

## Question #141: I've got a serious case of gym phobia. How can I get over it?

*The short answer:* The best strategy is to learn your way around at off-peak hours with the help of a trainer or gym veteran.

*If you're a newbie,* walking into a health club can be overwhelming, if not downright intimidating. At first glance, it probably seems like everyone in the joint has a Ph.D. in treadmill programming and has been hoisting barbells since infancy. In reality, clubs are constantly signing up new members, so you're not the only one who may be baffled by what the heck to do with a rope that's attached to a cable pulley.

Probably the best way to overcome any gym fears is to have a trainer or a knowledgeable friend show you the ropes. Try to work out when the club is nearly empty, like late morning, an hour before the gym closes, or early morning on a weekend. You can take your time noodling with the machinery without feeling the kind of pressure you might during peak time. Many clubs offer a complimentary training session when you sign up, so take advantage of the free expertise. You'll feel more at home in the gym once you know how to adjust the seats on the weight machines and have developed a workout plan. If you walk into the gym each day with a mission, you'll feel less self-conscious than if you roam around pondering which contraption to use next.

If you're more intimidated by the members of your gym than by the equipment, keep in mind that most people are too busy focusing on their own workouts to pay attention to what you or anyone else is doing. Most people are just there to work out, not check people out. And if you do have a question, most veterans will gladly demonstrate their intimate knowledge of, say, a triceps pressdown or a rear-delt fly machine. Often the size of a person's biceps is directly proportional to how helpful he or she will be.

Finally, you'll feel more comfortable once you get a handle on gym etiquette. Gyms have their own written and unwritten rules, like returning your dumbbells to the rack they came from, sharing the weight equipment if someone else is waiting (a.k.a. letting someone "work in" with you), and stepping aside at the drinking fountain if someone is waiting to take a sip while you're filling up your water bottle. All this stuff is pretty easy to pick up within a few workouts, and many gyms issue a "Be Fit Kit" containing their behavioral ten commandments. Before you know it, the gym will no longer seem like foreign territory.

# Strength Training: Sets, Reps, Routines, and Machines

Fact: Starting in your mid-thirties, you're likely to lose about one-third of a pound of muscle each year while gaining about a pound of fat. With muscle loss comes a drop in metabolism and, before you know it, the beginning of that dreaded "middle-age spread." By age 75, most people have lost at least one-third of their muscle mass, and two-thirds of all women can't lift 10 pounds — less than the weight of a bag of groceries. Nearly 30 percent of men age 75 and older can't make the lift. Many people in nursing homes are there due to lack of muscle mass.

What can you do to prevent this chain of events? Two words: Lift weights.

You might think that aerobic exercise is the key to staying slim and fit as you age, and it's true that jogging, cycling, and the like are essential for calorie burning and keeping your heart and lungs strong. But weight training can do for you what aerobic activities can't — namely, preserve your muscle mass, your strength, and your metabolism. Of course, pumping iron can also firm up your muscles and keep your bones healthy and, research suggests, may even help fight depression and reduce your risk of heart disease. All of this is a huge payoff for an activity that requires as little as 20 minutes twice a week.

In this section you'll find out how to get the greatest return on your investment in the weight room or home gym. We cover how often and how much weight you should lift, the pros and cons of various training techniques and types of equipment, plus everything you ever wanted to know about your abs.

Question #142: What's the difference between *resistance training, weight training,* and *strength training*?

*The short answer:* The terms are essentially synonymous.

*Anything that asks your muscles* to work against a force is a form of resistance. For instance, lifting a pile of newspapers provides resistance to your arms, shoulders, and upper back. When you pull back on your dog's leash to prevent him from running into the street, his body weight is a form of resistance, too.

When you are aiming to strengthen and tone your muscles, resistance usually comes in the form of a dumbbell or barbell, a stack of weight plates attached to a machine, a rubber exercise band, your own body weight, gravity, or some combination of all of these things. If they provide enough resistance, your muscles respond by developing strength. As your muscles get stronger, you need to challenge them with more resistance.

So really, weight training is just a form of resistance training, which is sometimes referred to as strength training. In this book, we use all three terms interchangeably.

Question #143: If I'm overweight, should I wait until I drop a few pounds before I begin lifting weights?

*The short answer:* No! In fact, lifting weights may actually help you lose weight, since it may boost your metabolism slightly.

*Sure, you lose weight by eating less* and burning more calories through cardiovascular exercise, but plenty of research suggests that adding weight training to the mix makes your weight-loss effort more effective. That's because weight training helps preserve your muscle mass — and therefore your metabolism. When you slim down using cardio exercise and diet alone, inevitably some of the weight you lose is muscle. You may lose some muscle even if you do add weight training to your program, but you'll lose a lot less this way (and maybe lose none or even gain muscle). Muscle tissue is much more active than fat, so when you have less muscle, your metabolism slows down slightly. Unless you cut even more calories and/or exercise more, it becomes difficult to continue losing weight or to keep it off.

Do be aware that when you take up weight training, the number on the scale may nudge upward a bit due to the increase in muscle mass. Unfortunately, some women become so alarmed at this increase that they swear off weightlifting. This is a big mistake. What matters is how much fat — not weight — you're losing. As we explain in Question #8, tracking changes in your body-fat percentage is a lot more useful than repeatedly stepping on the scale.

Regardless of what the scale says, you'll be happier with your weight-loss program if you include weight training because you'll look more toned. Losing weight through cardio exercise and diet can make you thinner, but it won't necessarily make you firmer.

## Question #144: How long does it take to gain a pound of muscle?

*The short answer:* It depends on your genetics and how hard you try. But in general, if you're a beginner lifting weights two or three times a week, it's possible to gain 1 pound of muscle per month for about six months. After that, muscle gain tends to slow down as the body adapts.

*There's no way to determine* how quickly any individual will gain a pound of muscle. Your genetic predisposition to build muscle plays a huge role. Mesomorphic body types (described in Question #17) tend to develop muscle faster than other body types, whereas ectomorphs struggle hardest to add muscle to their slim frames. Your progress also depends on how dedicated you are to your program. If you do little more than brush past the free weights on your way to and from the locker room, you're going to build muscle at a much slower rate than someone who lifts consistently.

## Question #145: Can I strengthen and tone my muscles with rubber exercise bands or tubes?

*The short answer:* Pulling on a rubber tube may not be the most macho of fitness endeavors, but research shows you can build a fair amount of strength this way.

*Bands and tubes are cheap,* portable, easy to use, and incredibly versatile. (Bands are thick and flat; tubes are, well, tubular, and typically have handles.) You can do literally hundreds of exercises with a $2 piece of rubber. The effectiveness of these exercises isn't entirely clear, since scientists aren't exactly lining up to research the benefits of rubber bands and tubing. Still, the handful of studies that do exist suggest that you can develop decent amounts of strength and muscle tone by using rubber-band resistance — over the course of a few months, perhaps as much strength as you can build from traditional weight training.

In the long run, though, bands have their limitations. We seriously doubt that any Mr. or Ms. Olympia winners got to the podium using rubber exercise bands as their primary form of resistance training. There are other good reasons why health clubs are stocked with chunks of steel and heavy machinery instead of bands and tubes. For one thing, it's difficult to gauge your progress with a tube or band since there are no measurements printed on them. Although you can adjust the resistance by choking up on the band or leaving more slack, you can't tell how much weight you're lifting, and with most bands it's impossible to know exactly where to grab hold so that you can equal the amount of resistance you used during your last workout. However, a clever new product called Band-a-line (available through performbetter.com) does come with demarcations for this purpose.

Also, some band exercises feel a bit choppy and awkward. This is because bands generate the greatest amount of resistance at the end of the movement, when they're completely stretched out. Unfortunately, your muscles' strength curve isn't likely to match up with the tension provided by the band. Most muscles are at their

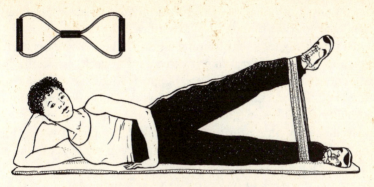

*Tubes (top) and resistance bands (above) are effective for building strength.*

strongest at the very beginning or somewhere in the middle of a movement, where the band provides the least resistance. Bands tend to work best for straightforward exercises like biceps curls and triceps extensions, where the bands move in a linear path instead of off to the side (as with a shoulder lateral raise) or in an arc-like path (as with a chest fly or pullover).

Although bands have their downside, the trade-offs are probably worth it if you're strapped for cash, don't have much room to exercise or store equipment, or don't want to lug around a suitcase full of dumbbells when you travel.

## Question #146: How many days a week should I lift weights?

*The short answer:* Ideally, you should work each major muscle group two or three times a week.

*If you work* your muscles less than two or three times a week, you won't build much strength. More than that is overkill; your muscles will be too fatigued to keep getting stronger. However, this rule doesn't limit you to two or three days in the weight room. If you really insist, you can lift weights every day of your life, as long as you target different muscle groups on different days. See Question #148 for details about "split routines."

Research suggests that training a muscle twice a week is pretty much as effective as training it three days a week, especially for beginners. The American College of Sports Medicine recommends that beginners start by lifting twice a week. Once they build some strength and develop their technique, they may see bigger improvements by lifting three days a week. Our opinion is that lifting two days a week is sufficient as long as you really put in the effort. In fact, many advanced lifters prefer hitting each muscle group twice a week in order to give their muscles enough rest between hard workouts.

## Question #147: Is there any benefit to lifting weights just once a week if that's all the time I have?

*The short answer:* Yes. Lifting once a week is better than nothing, although not nearly as effective as lifting two or three days a week.

*Consider a 12-week University of Alabama* study that compared two groups of experienced lifters. The groups did the same total amount of training — three sets of nine different exercises over the course of each week — but one group did all three sets of each exercise on a single day, whereas the other group did one set of each exercise three days a week. At the end of the study, the one-day group achieved about 62 percent of the strength gains of the three-day group.

The authors suspect that the reason for the difference in strength gains, despite equal training volume, is that a full week between training sessions allows time for muscles to atrophy. Some people start to lose training benefits after 96 hours, research suggests.

But the good news is, once you've developed a significant amount of strength from training two or three days a week, you'll be able to maintain it with just one training session per week for at least several months.

Question #148: My weight-training workouts seem to take forever. How do I keep myself from running out of steam?

*The short answer:* Try "functional training" — exercises that work several muscle groups at once — or try a split routine, a program that involves different muscles on different days.

*"Functional fitness"* is trainer-speak for training your body the way it operates in real life: Instead of doing moves that isolate a single muscle, you perform exercises that involve several muscles and joints. These moves mimic or enhance everyday and sports activities, forcing you to rely on your deeper musculature, your sense of balance, and your powers of concentration. A squat — which works your butt, thighs, back, and abdominal muscles — is a good example of a functional exercise. You use this movement every time you sit down, stand up, jump to spike a volleyball, sit astride a horse, bend to catch a ball, or any number of other common movements.

Performing a series of functional movements is not only great for your body, but also trims your training time because you don't have to hit each of your major muscle groups individually. If you choose the right moves — a trainer can help — you can get a decent workout with just four or five exercises.

If you're serious about strength training and have a schedule that lets you hit the weight room at least four days a week, another way to shorten each workout is to split your routine. With fewer muscle groups to target in any given workout session, you'll have more motivation and energy to give each exercise your all. You're likely to perform more sets per muscle group and use heavier weights than you would if you were working your entire body in a single session. Even if you do a split routine, make functional exercises part of your exercise lineup. Besides being timesavers, they're valuable for teaching your body to operate like a well-oiled machine rather than a series of moving parts.

When you do a split routine, you need to follow a sensible system rather than randomly choose the muscles you hit each workout. Most people follow one of two types of splits.

## Upper-Body/Lower-Body Split

You do all your upper-body exercises on one day and your lower-body moves on another. Abs and lower back can fit into either day of the split. Here's a sample schedule.

### Sample Schedule — Upper-Body/Lower-Body Split

| Day | Upper or Lower | Body Parts Exercised |
|-----|----------------|----------------------|
| 1 | Upper body | Chest, back, shoulders, triceps, biceps, abs |
| 2 | Lower body | Buttocks, quads, hamstrings, calves, lower back |
| 3 | | Rest |
| 4 | Upper body | Chest, back, shoulders, triceps, biceps, abs |
| 5 | Lower body | Buttocks, quads, hamstrings, calves, lower back |
| 6 | | Rest |
| 7 | | Rest |

## Complementary Muscle-Group Split

On each day, you work muscles that function as a team, like the chest and triceps or the back and biceps. Shoulders can fit into either upper-body day, since they're involved in just about every upper-body movement.

To save trips to the gym, you could add lower-body exercises to either of your upper-body workouts. The disadvantage to this schedule is that your workouts could grow longer than a made-for-TV movie on Lifetime. Some people take more rest days and simply cycle through the workouts in order. This means that every third week, you'd do one of the workouts only once. If you're lifting heavy weights, this isn't necessarily a bad thing. It'll give those muscle groups some extra rest. Here's a sample schedule.

## Sample Schedule — Complementary Muscle-Group Split

| Day | Body Parts Exercised |
| --- | --- |
| 1 | Chest, triceps, shoulders |
| 2 | Back, biceps, abs, lower back |
| 3 | Butt, quads, hamstrings, calves |
| 4 | Chest, triceps, shoulders |
| 5 | Back, biceps, abs, lower back |
| 6 | Butt, quads, hamstrings, calves |
| 7 | Rest |

## Question #149: Should I lift weights before or after my cardio workout?

*The short answer:* It depends on your priorities on a given day. In general, start your workout with the activity that you feel requires more of your energy that day.

*There's no hard-and-fast rule* about which type of exercise to do first. There are plenty of scenarios in which it makes more sense to start with cardiovascular exercise, and other cases in which you're better off hitting the weights when you're most fresh.

Let's say you do cardio exercise four days a week, and on two of those days you also lift weights. You want to make those lifting sessions really count, so on your lifting days, start with the weights (after a 5-minute cardio warm-up, of course). Follow these lifting sessions with easy-to-moderate cardio workouts, saving your tough cardio efforts for the days when you're not lifting.

On the other hand, if you have a relatively easy strength-training session planned (after, say, a tough session a couple of days earlier), go ahead and do your cardio first. No matter how hard you push, you probably won't compromise that easy lifting workout. (A cardio workout may compromise a more challenging lifting session.) Another option, for any day, is to split up your workout: Do 20 minutes of cardio, lift weights, and then do another 20 minutes of cardio. Or, do your lower-body strength exercises, do 30 minutes on the treadmill, and then do your upper-body routine.

You may go through phases in your training when building your cardio fitness is more important to you than developing strength, or vice versa. During those phases, you might want to start each workout with the activity that is your priority at the time. One final consideration: If you forgot to bring a towel to the gym, you'd better lift weights first, so that you don't leave the strength-training equipment drenched in your sweat!

## Question #150: Is one set of strength-training exercises as effective as three?

*The short answer:* It can be, if you are relatively new to strength training or you have modest goals and train three times a week. But if you dream of a body that any reality-TV contestant would be proud of, one set isn't going to cut it no matter how regularly you lift.

*There are some studies* suggesting that you can gain just as much strength performing one set as you can performing three, but the subjects in these studies lifted enormously heavy weights and gave 100 percent effort to each and every set. For beginners, this level of exertion isn't practical, since it's likelier to cause injury and the kind of muscle soreness that makes tying your shoes painful. And we think it's not a great idea to do super-heavy sets without at least one lighter warm-up set, anyway.

Other studies show that you can gain about two-thirds the strength with one set as you can with three sets, but only if you lift three days a week. When it comes to building moderate amounts of strength, most experts feel — and we agree — that how consistently you train is more important than the number of sets you do.

If you want significant results, you're better off doing three sets per muscle group per workout, assuming you lift two or three times a week. Bodybuilders, power lifters, and people aiming to transform their muscles into sculpted masterpieces typically add even more sets at some point in their training. Although performing 10 sets per muscle group probably will translate into more strength and tone, the extra benefits are probably too small to justify the extra time and effort for the average person.

## Question #151: If I'm doing multiple sets of an exercise, should I start with a light weight and build up, or should I go for a heavier weight while my muscles are fresh?

*The short answer:* Do a light set first.

*If you're aiming for maximum strength,* it might be tempting to start a set with a heavy weight while you're feeling fresh. But you'll actually be able to lift heavier — while keeping your injury risk low — if you warm up with one or two light sets before going for the gusto. A light set not only warms up your muscle fibers but also helps them "practice" the movement pattern. That's why you sometimes see guys with barrel-sized chests warming up on the bench press with nothing but the bar.

## Question #152: How long should I rest between sets?

*The short answer:* Like everything in weightlifting, the answer depends on your goals.

*Power lifters* and others aiming to build as much strength as possible often rest as long as five minutes between sets so their muscles can make a complete recovery. Those of us who don't aspire to lift a rhino overhead don't need to spend nearly as much time watching the clock between sets.

If you are a novice lifter, if you are recovering from an injury, or if you're lifting fairly heavy weights, take about 90 seconds before picking up a weight again. For the average person, this is plenty of time for a muscle to regroup. If you're more advanced and want to boost your workout intensity, limit your rest periods to 60 seconds. Your muscles won't quite recover from the last set, so they'll have to push harder to get through the workout.

To dial up the intensity of your weight workouts even more, cut your rest periods down to 30 seconds or less. This type of workout is a sort of hybrid between cardio and strength training; you won't be able to lift as much weight, but you'll sweat a whole lot more. For a real heart-pumping workout, try circuit training, a workout style that calls for moving quickly between exercises with little to no rest. We describe this type of training in Question #155.

### Question #153: How many repetitions of each strength-training exercise should I do?

*The short answer:* If you're a beginner, start by doing 15 reps per set, and after a month or so, increase your weights so that your muscles fatigue in the 8-to-12-rep range. Advanced lifters aiming for cantaloupe-sized biceps may want to perform fewer than 8 reps per set.

*To hear people in the weight room talk,* you'd think there was some complex algebraic function involved in determining the correct number of repetitions to perform per set. It's actually pretty simple: Determine your goals, and you've determined the number of reps you should do to achieve them. In general, the fewer reps you perform — using heavy enough weights that your muscles fatigue by the end of the set — the more size and strength you'll build. If you lift lighter weights and perform more reps, you'll develop less strength but more muscular endurance (the ability of a particular muscle to perform repetitive movements for a long time).

However, don't lighten the weights to the point where you can easily perform more than 15 reps. Programs that involve doing 100 leg lifts and 300 crunches are ineffective for developing muscle tone or even moderate strength. That's because any weight training set that lasts longer than about one minute isn't very effective for building strength. The maximum number of reps you can do in one minute using good form and moving at a careful, safe speed is about 15.

To reap the bone-density benefits of weight training, studies suggest that performing 6 to 12 reps is the optimal range. It's fine to stick with 15 reps when you do circuit training, a type of workout that involves moving quickly from one exercise to the next without much, if any, rest.

We don't recommend performing fewer than 8 reps unless you've already got a few months of lifting under your belt and are working toward developing maximum size and power. However, studies do suggest that for experienced lifters, dropping to 5 or 6 reps may be more effective for building strength than doing every workout in the 8-to-12 range. If you do embark on some heavy lifting, do it only for a few weeks at a time or mix it with lighter, higher-rep workouts. Your chances of injury and extreme soreness skyrocket when you push around very heavy weights.

## Question #154: What kind of weight-training program will give me tone without bulk?

*The short answer:* If you stay in the range of 8 to 12 repetitions — using weights heavy enough to challenge your muscles — you can rest assured that your muscles will become stronger and firmer without inflating you to NFL-linebacker proportions.

*Many women fear* that if they lift weights any heavier than a tube of hair gel, their muscles will become decidedly unfeminine. So they use dinky dumbbells and perform 20 to 30 repetitions, sometimes even more, on the assumption that a high-rep/low-weight program is the way to develop firm, defined muscles without developing the dreaded "bulk."

Reality check: Performing more than 15 reps is a big, fat waste of time. (We explain why in Question #153.) And even if you stay at the low end of the 8-to-15 range, you're about as likely to become bulky as you are to become independently wealthy selling ant farms. The vast majority of women just don't have enough testosterone to develop monster muscles. Even most men — try as they might — just don't have the genetics to look like Vin Diesel.

But what about those female bodybuilders with manly physiques? Well, they didn't get that way by accident. To develop that much size, they lift extremely heavy weights and spend long hours in the gym. They may do 30 sets for each muscle group and lift weights so heavy that they can only perform a couple of repetitions. And more than a few of them take steroids, in which case they also tend to sprout a beard, develop acne, and end up with a voice like the late Barry White's.

Also, bodybuilders have extremely (and often unhealthily) low levels of body fat, which makes their muscles look even larger.

How you respond to a weightlifting program depends in large part on your genetic predisposition toward building muscles. Certainly, some people build muscles more easily than others. Still, getting bulky is probably not something you need to worry about. In fact, for some people, developing even moderate muscle tone isn't easy. Performing dozens of reps with light weights certainly won't give you bulk, but that kind of program won't give you much of anything at all, except perhaps joint injuries from excessive repetition.

## Question #155: What exactly is circuit training, and is there any benefit to training this way?

*The short answer:* Circuit training is a fast-paced form of weight training that offers both strength and cardiovascular benefits. You move from one exercise to the next with little or no rest and then perform the "circuit" all over again.

*Why would anyone* want to dial up weight training to warp speed? To save time, for one thing. You can slam through a full-body routine, performing two or three sets per muscle group, in about 20 minutes. Plus, since you're constantly in motion, you can really get your heart pumping, reaping some aerobic benefits. You also burn more calories (about 8 per minute) than you would during a conventional weight routine (5 or 6 calories per minute).

Still, circuit training is a compromise. You won't build as much strength as you would with a traditional routine, because when you take minimal rest between sets, you can't lift as much weight. Your muscles don't have as much time to recover. Meanwhile, you won't get the same aerobic challenge as you would doing a straight-up cardio workout like a step class or treadmill jog. The only time you're actually moving fast is when you charge to the next exercise. For reasons we explain in Question #158, you still need to perform your repetitions slowly and with control.

Because circuit training is a compromise, we think it's best to reserve it for those times when you're in a hurry or need a change in your routine. You can circuit train for a month or so and then switch back to your typical routine, or you can use it once a week or so on a regular basis. At first you might need 30 seconds to catch your breath between exercises in a circuit, but as you build stamina, you'll be able to bounce from one move to the next with virtually no break. Just remember not to sacrifice good form for the sake of speed. And lighten your weights by one or two increments compared with your regular strength routine.

## Question #156: How do I know when I'm ready to lift heavier weights?

*The short answer:* Increase the weight when completing the last repetition of a set is no longer a challenge.

*Once you've established* the range of repetitions per set that you want to complete (see Question #153), chose a weight that challenges you for at least the minimum number of reps. Let's say you're aiming to do 10 repetitions for your biceps curls. This means you need to choose a weight that really fatigues your biceps by the 10th repetition. If you get to that 10th rep and feel like you could crank out a few more with good form, you're ready to move up to a heavier weight.

We recommend moving up by the smallest increment possible. Jumping up in weight too quickly can pose an injury risk. At the very least, you'll defeat the purpose of the exercise by relying on additional muscles to help you hoist the weight. Use too much weight with those biceps curls and you'll start rocking back and forth, using your lower back muscles to help hoist the dumbbells.

Get in the habit of paying attention to how your muscles feel at the end of each set, so you'll know when it's time to increase your weight. Many women — fearful that lifting heavier weights will give them monster muscles — make the mistake of sticking with weights that are too light long after they should have bumped it up. If you lift weights that aren't challenging enough, you're not going to get the strengthening or toning results you're looking for.

**Q**uestion #157: I'm curious to see how much weight I can possibly lift, but I'm not sure how many plates to put on the bar. Is there an accurate way to estimate my "max"?

*The short answer:* Use the table on page 207 to estimate your max based on the number of repetitions you can perform with a lighter weight.

*"What's your max?"* That's a question that serious weightlifters like to ask each other, the same way marathon runners ask, "What's your PR?" — your personal record — or golfers ask, "What's your handicap?" It's only natural to want to know just how fast, skilled, or strong you are. Your "max," also known as your "1-rep max," is the heaviest amount of weight that you can lift one time for a particular exercise. Typically, lifters are curious to know their 1-rep max on heavy-duty exercises like the bench press or the squat.

Choosing a target weight can be tricky. If you aim too high, of course, you will fail at the attempt and may wrench a muscle or tendon in the process. But if you're too conservative, you'll lose out on the glory of finding your true max. And coming *near* your max may leave you too pooped to make another attempt at a heavier weight.

The commonly used chart at right can help you find a reasonable target weight.

To use the table, you first need to know the number of reps that you can perform with a weight that is lighter than your max. Let's say that with 90 pounds loaded on the bench press, you can do 10 repetitions — and not one more. (For the table to work, this must be 10 reps to absolute "failure.") Check the table and find the percentage associated with that number of repetitions. Now divide 90 by .75. The result — 120 pounds — is your estimated 1-rep max.

### Estimating Your 1-Rep Max

| Reps | % of 1-rep max |
|------|----------------|
| 1 | 100 |
| 2 | 95 |
| 3 | 90 |
| 4 | 88 |
| 5 | 86 |
| 6 | 83 |
| 7 | 80 |
| 8 | 78 |
| 9 | 76 |
| 10 | 75 |
| 11 | 72 |
| 12 | 70 |

Keep in mind that these percentages are just estimates, and they may work better for some exercises than others. Also, how confident you're feeling and how well rested you are can play a big role in whether you succeed at a certain lift. Whether you've warmed up enough may also affect your lift. Before attempting a max, do at least two warm-up sets with lighter weights.

Don't try to max out unless you've been lifting weights for at least a few months and have a lot of experience with that particular exercise. You don't want to try a bench press max your first day in the gym when you can't even keep the bar from wobbling. And even then, don't try it more than once every three or four weeks. Experienced lifters tend to make strength gains at a slow pace, so there's no point in testing yourself too often. Finally, be sure you've enlisted a "spotter" for your max attempt, someone who is standing by with hands poised to grab the bar just in case your muscles fail to cooperate.

**Question #158: I've heard that the Super Slow method of weight training is more effective than lifting weights at a normal speed. Is this true?**

*The short answer:* Zooming through your reps is clearly a bad idea, because you rely on momentum rather than muscle power. However, the jury is out on whether Super Slow training — a technique that involves taking a full 10 to 45 seconds to lift a weight and then another 10 to 45 seconds to lower it — is more effective for building strength than the traditional pace of 2 seconds up and 4 seconds down.

*Super Slow training* has made a media splash in recent years, in large part because of sensational claims by its proponents that have nothing to do with building strength. Among the claims: Aerobic exercise is both useless and dangerous, and Super Slow training alone is the best way to lose weight.

Given the hundreds upon thousands of studies showing the benefits of aerobic exercise and the complete absence of published research in support of Super Slow as a weight-loss method, most exercise experts dismiss these claims outright. Super Slow proponents dismiss these experts right back, maintaining that the Everest-sized mountain of published research was conducted by inept investigators using flawed or fabricated data. In fact, the founder of the Super Slow Exercise Guild, an organization of Super Slow proponents, says on the group's Web site (superslow.com) that he considers exercise physiologists to be not scientists but rather "glorified coaches, nothing more."

If you cut through the inflammatory language and personal attacks, is there any merit at all to Super Slow training? We think that, purely as a strength-building technique, there just might be something to this method of training. Certainly, slowing down your repetitions makes your muscles work harder. And when you eliminate momentum, you're not likely to put your joints or muscles at risk by swinging around weights that are too heavy. The technique is so darned hard that it forces you to use weights that you can control.

Still, only a handful of studies have been conducted on Super Slow training, so the strength benefits aren't clear. One study compared a modified Super Slow program (10 seconds lifting, 4 seconds lowering) with a traditional program (2 seconds lifting, 1 second pause, 4 seconds lowering). Both groups did one set of each exercise, but the Super Slow group did 4 to 6 repetitions while the traditional group did 10 to 12 reps. After 10 weeks, the slow lifters had gained 50 percent more strength than the other group.

Another study, done at the University of Alabama at Birmingham, found that Super Slow burns 45 percent fewer calories than some other traditional resistance training methods. The study also found that Super Slow didn't elevate post-workout metabolism for as long as other strength-training methods did.

We think Super Slow is worth trying if you're looking to improve the size and strength of your muscles — perhaps if you're stuck on a plateau and want to try something new. It's also an option to consider if you want to save time, since Super Slow training calls for performing just one set of each exercise (although it's certainly a long set that requires patience to complete).

Just know that Super Slow isn't for everyone. Beginners may find its muscle-ripping intensity too much to handle and even weightlifting vets may experience excruciating muscle soreness after the first few sessions. If you do enjoy this technique, just don't count on it to melt away pounds or replace your cardio workouts.

## Question #159: Will weight training make me muscle-bound?

*The short answer:* No, that's just a myth.

*There's a persistent rumor* that lifting weights makes your muscles so tight that you can barely bend your arm enough to scratch your nose. But research shows that weight training actually makes you more flexible, as long as you complete what exercise scientists call the "full range of motion." This means moving through the exercise as far as your muscles and the joints can comfortably and safely go, rather than cutting a movement short (or pushing it too far).

If you repeatedly stop short, it's possible to wind up feeling tight, but only if your muscles are on the tight side to begin with and only if you use poor form over a long period of time. (But don't move too far, either — you risk overstretching your ligaments and causing injury.) Every muscle, every joint, and every exercise has its own ideal range of motion. If you stay within that range, you'll not only have no worries about compromised flexibility, you'll probably become even more flexible.

## Question #160: Does it really matter what order I do my strength exercises in?

*The short answer:* In general, yes. You should work your larger muscles before working any smaller muscles that assist them.

*When you work your larger muscle groups,* such as your back, chest, and butt, the exercises typically require assistance from smaller muscle groups. For instance, when you do a lat pulldown — an exercise that focuses primarily on the latissimus dorsi muscles of your middle back — your biceps and shoulders also kick in, helping the lats as you pull the bar down to your chest. If you were to tire out your biceps and shoulders before performing this exercise, you wouldn't be able to use as much weight for the lat pulldown, and your lats would get short shrift.

Don't worry about those smaller muscles getting too pooped from their assistant duties. Since they're only helping, they should have plenty of gas left when they take center stage. Assisting the larger muscles is like a warm-up for them. You'll still get a quality biceps workout after you're done working your lats.

This largest-to-smallest muscle rule applies only to exercises within each zone of the body. For the most part, your upper-body muscles aren't involved in lower-body lifts and vice versa, so you don't need to worry about exercising, say, your chest (a large mus-

cle group) before your calves (a small group). Although it's important to work the muscles within each zone — upper body, middle body, and lower body — from largest muscle to smallest, you
can work the three zones in any order you want.

Here's a rundown of the muscle groups, from largest to smallest, within each zone. When two muscle groups are on the same
line, this means you can work either of them first.

**The Three Muscle-Group Zones**

| Upper Body | Lower Body | Middle Body |
|---|---|---|
| Middle back (lats), chest | Buttocks | Rectus abdominis |
| | Quadriceps, hamstrings | Obliques |
| Shoulders | Inner thighs, outer thighs | Lower back |
| Biceps, triceps | | |
| Wrists | Calves | |

## Question #161: How often should I vary my weight workout?

*The short answer:* If you're looking to build a modest amount of
strength and muscle tone, you can probably get by with doing the
same routine forever. However, if you want to keep improving —
and keep from getting bored — you're better off overhauling your
routine every few months or even from workout to workout.

*Unless you're talking* about, say, global warming, change is usually for the good. This notion applies to strength training, too. If
you're new to lifting, research shows, pretty much any program
will keep you improving for the first three to four months. But
after that, people who vary their routines tend to show significantly more improvement than those who do the same old, same
old. Exercise scientists have a fancy name for the concept of periodic change: periodization.

The classic model of periodization typically involves breaking
up your training into four- to eight-week phases, each with a particular purpose. In the first phase, you might do several sets per

muscle group, performing 12 to 15 repetitions per set. In the next phase, you might drop the number of sets, increase your weights, and perform 8 to 10 reps per set. You might devote the third phase to lifting even heavier weights, performing 6 to 8 reps. Your last phase might be a recovery phase: You might do a light workout just once a week. Studies show that this form of periodization does an excellent job of building maximum strength and getting you ready for sports such as football, basketball, sprinting, and tennis. Results seem to be especially good when training phases last longer than four weeks.

Another effective method of periodization is called "undulating." Like a wave, your training volume constantly rises and falls. With this method, you cycle through different workouts over the course of a week or ten days. For instance, on Monday you might lift heavier weights and aim for 8 reps. On Wednesday you might use more moderate weights and perform 12 reps. Friday might be more of a recovery day; you could do some fast-paced circuit training, doing 15 reps with lighter weights and no rest between sets.

In addition to changing the number of sets and reps you perform, it's also smart to periodically change your exercises. Instead of doing your usual dumbbell chest press, do the exercise on an incline or decline bench; instead of doing the leg press machine, do squats. Working your muscles from different angles helps stimulate them to get stronger and keeps your workout routine from being, well, routine.

Q**uestion #162: I've heard that breathing technique is important when you lift weights. When should I inhale and when should I exhale?**

*The short answer:* In most cases, the best pattern is to exhale through your mouth when you exert an effort and inhale through your nose when you release the effort.

*This breathing pattern* ensures that your muscles get an optimal supply of oxygen, via your lungs and then bloodstream, to help fuel your lift. It also helps you maintain a steady rhythm as you perform your repetitions. Consider the shoulder press, an exercise that involves pushing dumbbells (or a barbell) overhead from shoulder height. Pressing the weights upward is the toughest part of the lift, so that's when you exhale forcefully through your mouth, pushing the air from your diaphragm. Lowering the weights is the easiest part of the lift, so this is when you inhale deeply through your nose, drawing in plenty of oxygen for the next repetition. When the oxygen enters your bloodstream, the oxygen-rich blood floods into the muscles, providing them with more energy for the lift. Don't forget to inhale before your first repetition.

If you're a beginning lifter, breathing in the proper sequence may be too much to think about. In that case, don't worry about it, and just breathe in whatever sequence comes naturally. The important thing is simply to remember to breathe, something many novices forget about. As you gain experience, the proper breathing pattern is something you'll be able to work on.

There is one exception to the breathing pattern we've described. If you're performing extremely heavy lifts — if, say, you're lifting so much weight that you can perform only one or two repetitions — most experts recommend holding your breath during the effort and exhaling in a short, deep burst when releasing. In this case, holding your breath creates extra pressure within your abdominal region, which serves as protection for your lower back and diaphragm. However, holding your breath also causes a sharp spike and then quick drop in blood pressure, which can lead to fainting and, in extreme cases, a heart attack. For this reason, this breathing technique is best left to veterans such as power lifters.

## Question #163: What's the difference between barbells and dumbbells, and what are the pros and cons of each?

*The short answer:* Barbells are the long bars that you see Olympic weightlifters and characters on TV prison dramas hoisting overhead with both hands. Dumbbells are the shorter versions that

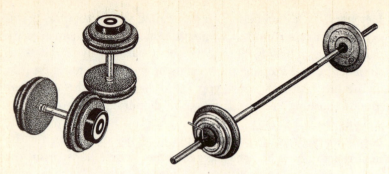

*Free weights are versatile and inexpensive.*

you can lift with one hand. (And no, you're not a dumbbell for asking.)

*Dumbbells and barbells* are considered "free weights" because they are not connected to any cables or pulleys or other machinery. For many exercises, you can use either barbells or dumbbells. For instance, you can lie on a bench and press up a barbell (hence the name of this exercise, the bench press), or you can do virtually the same movement using two dumbbells (in which case the exercise is called the dumbbell chest press). You can do the squat with a bar sitting on your shoulders, behind your neck, or with a dumbbell in each hand, either down by your sides or up on your shoulders.

Both dumbbells and barbells have their advantages. Dumbbells are especially useful for beginners because they come as light as 1 pound, whereas at most health clubs the lightest barbell you'll find weighs about 20 pounds. (However, you may come across lighter, foam-padded barbells called Body Bars, which range from 8 to 24 pounds. These are more popular for body-sculpting classes or home use.) The bar that sits on the bench press rack typically weighs 45 pounds.

Another advantage to dumbbells is that they allow each arm to work independently. When you do the bench press, for instance, your stronger side may do a disproportionate amount of the work. But the dumbbell chest press forces your weaker side to carry its own weight. For home exercisers, dumbbells may be a better investment than barbells because you can use them for a greater variety of exercises.

But barbells have their benefits, too. You can generally lift more total weight using one barbell than you can two dumbbells, so if you're aiming for maximum strength, barbell exercises can really help. For instance, when squatting, it can be difficult to use perfect technique while holding a heavy dumbbell in each hand. Typically you can handle a lot more weight — thereby giving your lower body a much greater challenge — with a barbell across your shoulders.

## Question #164: How do I know when I'm ready to graduate from weight machines to free weights?

*The short answer:* Actually, weight machines aren't something you graduate from, like high school or a red belt in karate. Weight machines and free weights are appropriate for beginners and advanced lifters alike, and the best workouts combine both types of equipment.

*It's true that weight machines* have many benefits for rookies. For one, they have built-in safety features. Because most weight machines move in a predetermined pathway, a novice can use them with minimal instruction and minimal risk of performing an exercise incorrectly. It takes more practice to master good form using dumbbells and barbells. Also, as long as you keep your fingers away from the stack of weight plates, there's no risk that any chunks of steel will come crashing down on your body parts.

All that said, beginners shouldn't be afraid to use free weights. Most free-weight exercises don't require tremendous amounts of strength or coordination, and they're plenty safe as long as you use an appropriate amount of weight. Plus, they have some distinct advantages over machines. For instance, free-weight exercises generally require you to use several muscle groups simultaneously, the way you do in everyday life. For example, when you use the biceps curl machine, the majority of your muscles sit idle while you bend and straighten your arms. But when you do standing biceps curls with dumbbells or a barbell, your abdominal and lower back muscles kick in to stabilize your body while you exercise your arms.

What's more, free-weight exercises allow your joints and muscles to move in ways that may be more comfortable for your particular body. When you use the shoulder press machine, you can adjust the seat height and your grip on the handles, but that's it; you're locked into the up-and-down motion set by the machine. If you happen to be too short or too tall for the machine, that's your tough luck. On the other hand, you can do the dumbbell shoulder press in either a sitting or a standing position. Plus, you have the freedom to position the weights a tiny bit forward, backward, out to the side, or however your body is most comfortable.

Another benefit of free weights: You can do more exercises with them. There's not a heckuva lot you can do with a hamstring curl machine other than hamstring curls (although we suppose you could use the contraption as extra seating for a Super Bowl party). But with a pair of dumbbells, you can literally do dozens, if not hundreds, of exercises, working your muscles from countless angles.

For home exercisers, free weights are usually the best options due to space and financial limitations. Even a multigym — a machine that combines many exercise machines into one frame — costs at least $1,000 and will hog a sizable portion of your den. You can purchase a whole array of free weights for a few hundred dollars or less. Several sets of dumbbells and a bench take up a fraction of the room consumed by a machine.

So if free weights are so fabulous, why would advanced lifters have any use for machines? Because certain key movements just aren't possible with dumbbells and barbells. For back exercises such as the lat pulldown (pulling a bar down to your chest) or the seated row (which mimics the motion of pulling oars through the water), there simply is no free-weight equivalent. Although there are several effective back exercises you can perform with dumbbells or barbells, you can't hit all the angles you can while using some type of machinery.

Also, no matter what your fitness level, machines can save you time. Adding weight plates to a barbell can eat up a fair amount of time, especially if you're changing the weight for each set. You can move quickly from machine to machine without making too many adjustments.

### Question #165: Why is the crunch better than the old-fashioned sit-up?

*The short answer:* Because the crunch forces your abs to work harder and is safer for your lower back.

*Sitting up all the way* — touching your elbows to your knees the way you used to in phys ed — doesn't require much effort on the part of your abdominals. The muscles that do the most work are your hip flexors, a set of strong, tight muscles that run from your upper thighs to your pelvis. When you overemphasize these muscles, they get stronger, shorter, and tighter.

The last thing most of us need is stronger and tighter hip flexors. When these muscles get too tight and strong, especially when compared with your abdominals and lower back muscles, they tug downward on your pelvis, causing your lower back to overarch and your butt to stick out. This poor posture also increases your propensity for lower back pain. Hooking your feet under a couch or having a friend hold them down only exacerbates the situation. With your feet locked in place, the movement is generated almost exclusively from your hip flexors.

A crunch may look wimpier than a full sit-up because you lift your torso just a few inches off the ground, but this limited movement actually puts your abs in action. You stop curling upward before the hip flexors take over. You can minimize hip-flexor involvement even further by doing crunches with your legs lifted off the floor. Start with your legs bent. As your abs get stronger, you can hold your legs in a straighter position.

## Question #166: Is the crunch the best way to work your abs?

*The short answer:* No. For all we said in the previous question about the benefits of the crunch compared with the full sit-up, this exercise isn't especially effective compared with many other moves you can do to strengthen your middle.

*Several studies have tested* the effectiveness of abdominal moves by hooking electrodes to various points of the subjects' abs, then measuring the electrical activity of the muscles during exercise. The more electricity produced, the more muscle fibers used. These studies, including one sponsored by the nonprofit American Council on Exercise and conducted at San Diego State University, found that the crunch falls toward the bottom of the list of effective ab exercises (along with three exercises performed using abdominal infomercial gizmos). At least a dozen other simple abdominal moves fared better. One of the most highly rated was the ball crunch, shown on pages 220 and 221. (See the chart on page 219 for a complete list.)

These exercises are particularly effective because they engage all of your abdominal muscles at once, forcing them to work together the way they do in everyday life. For instance, performing the crunch on a physioball requires tensing your entire midsection to keep you from rolling off the ball, so you're involving significantly more muscle fibers than when you do a crunch on the floor. In general, exercises that involve a lot of stabilization — holding your body still — and work multiple abdominal muscle groups will give you the strongest, firmest middle.

Exercises such as the traditional floor crunch work primarily one abdominal muscle, but you actually have four abdominal muscle groups. The *rectus abdominis* is the large thin sheet of muscle that runs the length of your torso from the top of your rib cage to your pelvis. Its job is to bend you forward from the middle and, more importantly, to keep the center of your body still and stable when you move other parts of your body. The *internal*

## The Best and Worst Ab Exercises

The following abdominal exercises were ranked best (1) to worst (13) by a San Diego State University study, based on how well they worked the rectus abdominis, the main abdominal muscle.

| Ranking | Exercise | How It's Done |
| --- | --- | --- |
| 1 | Bicycle | While lying on your back, twist from the middle and bring your opposite elbow to your opposite knee. |
| 2 | Captain's chair | Place your back against the padding of a captain's chair (see the illustration on page 221) and raise your knees to your chest. |
| 3 | Ball crunch | Lie with your back on an exercise ball and perform a traditional crunch. |
| 4 | Vertical leg crunch | Lie on your back with your legs straight up in the air. Lower them a small way and then raise them back up. |
| 5 | Torso Track | Get on the Torso Track machine face-down and grasp the handles. Use the apparatus to guide you. |
| 6 | Long-arm crunch | Do a basic crunch with your arms extended behind your head. |
| 7 | Reverse crunch | Lie on your back with your feet off the floor and your knees bent. Roll your buttocks off the floor to curl your knees toward your middle, then lower. |
| 8 | Crunch with heel push | Get into a basic crunch position with your heels lifted and your toes up. Every time you crunch upward, push your heels into the floor. |
| 9 | Ab Roller | Lie on your back with your arms pressed into the frame of an Ab Roller machine. Use the motion of the machine to roll you upward into a crunch and then lower you to the start. |
| 10 | Hover | With your back straight, balance on your elbows and the balls of your toes. Hold this position as long as possible. |
| 11 | Traditional (basic) crunch | Lie on your back with your hands behind your head, elbows bent, feet flat on the floor. Curl your head, neck, and shoulder blades up off the floor and lower to the start. |
| 12 | Exercise tube pull | Tie an exercise tube to a doorknob or other sturdy object. Lie on the floor with your head toward the tube and grasp one end in each hand. As you crunch, pull the tube with you. |
| 13 | Ab Rocker | Sit in the chair of the Ab Rocker machine and twist and rotate your middle. |

and *external obliques* wrap around your sides from front to back; besides generating twisting and bending movements, they act along with your other ab muscles as sort of a girdle to protect your lower back during other movements. The *transversus abdominis* muscles reside beneath your *rectus abdominis,* so you can't see or feel them. They function only during strong exhalation and when you stabilize your body.

### Ball Crunch (2 or 3 sets, 8 to 15 reps)

A. Lie on your back on top of a physioball so that your entire torso is resting on the curve of the ball and your feet are flat on the floor about hip width apart. Place your hands behind your head without lacing your fingers together. Keep your elbows wide but rounded slightly inward. Tilt your chin back to align your neck with the rest of your spine.

B. Exhale and curl your head, neck, and shoulders up and forward. Hold a moment and lower.

Tips: To make this exercise more challenging, bring your feet closer together or lift one foot up off the floor. To make this exercise easier, spread your feet slightly wider or use a spotter to help you with your balance.

*A*

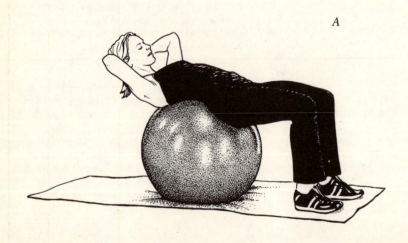

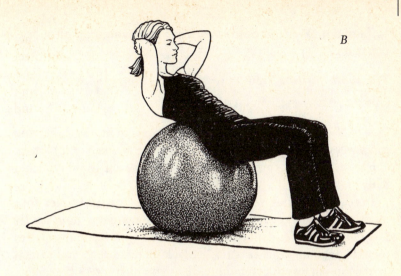

*B*

Here's how the exercises rank for strengthening the obliques.

1. Captain's chair
2. Bicycle
3. Reverse crunch
4. Hover
5. Vertical leg crunch
6. Ball crunch
7. Torso Track
8. Crunch with heel push
9. Long-arm crunch
10. Ab Roller
11. Traditional (basic) crunch
12. Exercise tube pull
13. Ab Rocker

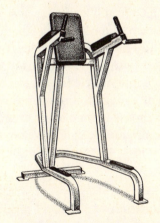

*Knee raises on the captain's chair do a great job of targeting the abs.*

## Question #167: Should I work my abs every day or every other day?

*The short answer:* Train your abdominal muscles two or three days a week.

*One of the most widely held misconceptions* in fitness is that you can never exercise your abdominal muscles too much or too often. Consequently, some people slam out 100 or even 1,000 crunches daily.

In reality, training your abs every day is a waste of time. Your main ab muscle group, the rectus abdominis, is predominantly fast-twitch muscle (defined in Question #19). It responds best to focused, high-intensity training — the kind that brings you to near exhaustion in less than a minute. If you do high-intensity training every day, you will break down your muscles rather than strengthen them. They never have a chance to rebuild and get stronger. You'll get better, faster results by working your abs the same way you train your other muscles: doing two or three sets of 8 to 12 repetitions to fatigue, two or three times a week.

It's key to work your abs from different angles, so that you involve more muscle fibers, and to perform exercises that are challenging enough to tire your muscles by the end of each set. Rather than choose the mundane crunch, for instance, perform crunches on a physioball, which are considerably tougher. Then give your abs at least 48 hours to rest between workouts.

## Question #168: Can I reduce my love handles by twisting or bending side to side?

*The short answer:* No. Twisting from side to side does not reduce fat and is unsafe for your lower back.

*Just as abdominal exercises* won't flatten your belly and the Thigh-Master won't slim your thighs, side twists and bends won't reduce your waistline. You simply can't target an area with repetitive exercise and expect the fat to melt away. Where you lose fat has more to do with genetics than anything else; we're all preprogrammed to gain and lose in specific áreas, in a specific order. Forget about twisting side to side and spend the time on some calorie-burning exercise like running, walking, cycling, or skating. Regular exercise, in combination with watching what you eat, is the most effective way to shed body fat. And while there is no guarantee where you will lose the fat, there's a very good chance that at least some of it will come off your love handles.

If twists and bends won't reduce your love handles, will they at least firm up the muscles underneath? Not really. Your obliques, a group of abdominal muscles that wrap around your middle like a girdle, get only a minimal benefit from these exercises. Twists don't require your obliques to work against much resistance or against gravity (which is just another form of resistance), so they don't offer much strength or tone. They can, however, wrench your lower back. One of the places the obliques are anchored is your lower spine. Twisting vigorously tugs on these muscles, which, in turn, tug on the spine — not an ideal scenario for an area that's fragile to begin with.

The two exercises shown on pages 224 and 225 are far more effective for your obliques than twists and bends. Targeting the obliques is important because, more than any other abdominal group, they anchor your lower spine. Stronger obliques go a long way toward minimizing back pain and improving posture.

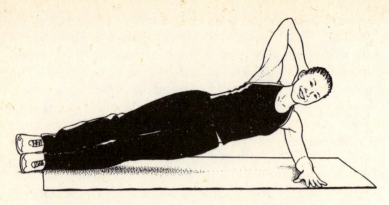

## Side Plank (2 or 3 sets of 3 or 4 reps on each side)

A. Lie on your side, propped up on your forearm with your legs out straight, hips stacked directly on top of each other. Pull your abs in and place your hand across your body or on your hip.

B. Balancing on the bottom edge of the foot that's on the floor and on your forearm, press your body up off the floor, keeping it as straight and balanced as possible. Hold for at least 10 slow counts. Between reps, drop down for a few seconds to rest.

Tips: To make this exercise harder, try lifting your free arm over your head. To make it easier, balance on your calf instead of your foot.

## Bicycle (2 or 3 sets of 8 to 15 reps on each side)

A. Lie on your back with your hands behind your head. Don't lace your fingers together. Round your elbows slightly inward. Bend your knees and lift your feet off the floor so that your thighs are perpendicular to the floor.

B. Extend your left leg straight up and out at a 45-degree angle to the floor as you lift your upper body and twist your left shoulder toward your right knee. Hold a moment, then twist to the other side so that your right leg is straight and your right shoulder twists toward your bent left knee. Complete all reps before lowering to the floor.

Tips: To make this exercise harder, don't lift your straightened leg quite as high. To make it easier, don't straighten your leg all the way.

*A*

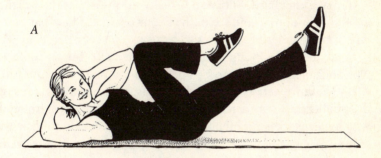

*B*

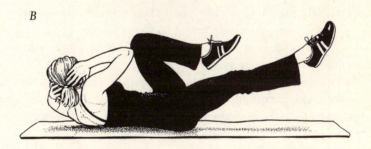

## Question #169: Are body-sculpting classes a good way to firm up?

*The short answer:* They can be quite effective, as long as the instructor follows the basic rules of strength training. But if the rules are flouted — with weights that are too light or exercises performed in the wrong order — you may be wasting your time.

*Maybe it's the decibel level of the music* or the spandex outfits squeezing the common sense out of the instructor, but some body-sculpting instructors toss the basic laws of strength training right out the window. Especially common are violations of the "rep rule" — the consensus, among exercise experts, that you should perform 8 to 15 repetitions per set using a reasonably challenging weight. Some body-sculpting instructors perform dozens, if not hundreds, of reps of a single exercise. This may make you feel like you're working hard, but what it really means is that the weights are too light to tone and strengthen your muscles. Plus, that many repetitions can lead to injuries.

Some body-sculpting instructors also make the mistake of working smaller muscle groups before larger ones. (See Question #160 for more details about why this is a problem.) As a result, the smaller muscles are too pooped to help out the larger muscles, which means the larger muscles won't get to work up to their potential. For instance, an instructor might lead you in a series of shoulder exercises and then have you pop down on the floor to attempt a set of pushups for the larger chest muscles. Of course, you wouldn't be able to do as many pushups as you could if your shoulder muscles were fresh. Plus, you might feel a twinge in your shoulder joint from overwork.

When evaluating a body-sculpting class, keep in mind that the rules of strength training remain the same whether you're on your own operating machines in a gym or doing an exercise-band routine set to music with a room full of people.

Some body-sculpting instructors really know what they're doing, and if you can locate these people, you can learn a lot from them. You can pick up new exercises or variations on old ones and learn how to use different equipment — such as bands, balls, and Body Bars — that you might not otherwise go near. A body-sculpting class can also be a good, inexpensive way to get professional instruction, especially if you can't afford a personal trainer on a regular basis. Taking a class can also help you dig yourself out of a training rut, and if you can't muster the motivation to lift weights solo, the energy of a group class can be highly motivating.

# Question #170: Should I wear a weight belt when pumping iron?

*The short answer:* No. Research suggests that weight belts offer no benefit. People with a history of heart disease or high blood pressure should steer especially clear of this accessory.

*Lifters who wear belts* do so in the belief that it will protect their lower back, especially during heavy-duty exercises such as squats, overhead presses, and bench presses. The theory is that the belt will act like a corset, compressing and stabilizing the lower back muscles so they're less likely to get overextended. As a result, the theory goes, you can push around heavy weights without having to worry about wrenching your back.

Although this may make sense intuitively, research has not supported this theory. In fact, after surveying 30 years of research, the National Institute for Occupational Safety and Health chose not to recommend belts for workers involved in heavy lifting because of a lack of scientific evidence showing a benefit. In a two-year study of Wal-Mart employees, for instance, researchers found no difference in reports of back pain between workers who wore belts every day and those who never or rarely used them.

Although scientists have not compared injury rates among belt-using and beltless weightlifters, there's no reason to believe weight belts would protect people lifting heavy barbells any more than they would help those hoisting 32-inch TV sets. What's more, many experts suspect, belts may even be detrimental in the weight room. Some studies show that wearing a belt takes work away from your abdominal and lower back muscles. If these muscles don't increase in strength in proportion to your other muscles, your lower back may be more susceptible to injury.

Although there's scant research on the effect of weight belts on back-injury risk, plenty of studies show that wearing a belt causes a significant increase in pressure within your abdominal wall as you exert an effort to lift a weight. You always build up a certain amount of this "intra-abdominal pressure" when you lift, but the belt increases it even further. This happens even when you lift relatively light weights and leads to sharper increases in blood pressure. If you have high blood pressure or a history of heart disease, your blood pressure may skyrocket to potentially dangerous levels.

## Question #171: Is it safe for kids to lift weights?

*The short answer:* Yes, as long as the kids are supervised and keep the weights on the lighter side.

*Lifting weights* won't turn your child into a mini-muscleman, nor will it stunt his growth, weaken his bones, or damage his muscles. The American Academy of Pediatrics and other professional organizations give the green light for children as young as 7 to pump iron.

That doesn't mean your child should take up power lifting or try to "max out" on the bench press. Experts recommend that kids do one or two sets for each muscle group, performing 8 to 15 repetitions per set using relatively light weights. Unlike adults, they shouldn't push to fatigue on the last rep. Kids who lift should do so two or three times a week and should also be supervised at all times by an experienced adult.

Kids definitely get stronger from weightlifting, but they don't typically gain size until after they reach puberty. This is because they don't have enough muscle-building hormones coursing through their bloodstreams. Most of their strength gains are due to improved connections between their muscles and brains rather than brawnier muscle fibers.

Strength training won't necessarily give your kid the edge in sports, although research suggests it may help him or her recover faster from an injury and will certainly help improve balance and coordination. And considering the skyrocketing levels of childhood obesity, encouraging your child to do any sort of physical activity that doesn't involve a mouse or a joystick can only be a good thing.

# Getting Your Money's Worth: Fitness Equipment, Gadgets, and Trainers

There are plenty of smart purchases you can make to help in your quest for a firmer, trimmer body, whether it's a few sessions with a certified personal trainer, a quality Spin bike, or a decently priced gym membership. The right equipment or environment can inspire you, challenge you, and help you reach your goals. But for all the great deals and nifty gizmos available, there's also plenty of schlock.

This section is for anyone who has ever wondered, "Can that electrical stimulation gizmo really zap fat off my middle?" or "Are those Bowflex contraptions any good?" It's for anyone who has ever walked into a Foot Locker and been baffled by the rows upon rows of athletic shoes, thinking, "How the heck am I supposed to choose one?"

This section will help you become a savvy consumer so that no matter what your budget or space requirements, you won't wind up with a basement full of junk you can't even unload on eBay.

## Question #172: What should I look for when I buy athletic shoes?

*The short answer:* Forget about the swishes and stripes. Pick shoes designed for your most frequent activity, your feet, and your biomechanics. Don't even think about breaking them in; athletic shoes should be comfortable from the get-go.

*Kevlar, cantilevers,* ClimaCool Response Cushions — athletic shoe jargon is confusing enough to make you want to turn on your heel and bolt out of the store. But finding the right shoe isn't all that complicated if you understand a few basic facts about your feet.

Any activity you do more than twice a week on a regular basis deserves a dedicated shoe. This may sound like a marketing gimmick, but you do use your feet in different ways for different types of exercise. For example, when you walk, your heel strikes the ground first, which is why walking shoes are heavily padded at the heel. Running shoes have substantial heel padding, too, but are more flexible from head to toe since your foot bends a lot more when you run. Aerobic shoes have firmer ankle support and are less bendy than walking shoes. They're engineered to provide plenty of stability for jumping, stepping, and sideways movements.

Also consider: Are your feet wide or narrow? Do you have high arches or collapsed arches? If your arches are flat, look for shoes that offer extra arch support. If your feet tend to supinate (roll excessively outward), look for a shoe with extra "motion control" — in other words, one that keeps your foot stable and centered in the shoe as you move. If your feet overpronate (roll excessively inward) look for a shoe that offers extra cushioning, motion control, and shock absorption.

Overweight exercisers and anyone with a history of injuries, such as chronic knee pain or weak ankles, should buy shoes with extra cushioning to help support their weight and protect their joints. Lighter, pain-free exercisers can probably get away with less substantial shoe models.

Always try on shoes with athletic socks, and do it at the end of the day, when your feet are at their most swollen. Take a test run to make sure no parts rub and your longest toe doesn't bump up against the front of the shoe. Some stores keep a treadmill in the shoe department for test drives. We suggest shopping at a store that specializes in athletic shoes because the staffers tend to be more educated and helpful. Once you nail down shoes you're happy with, you can save a ton of money buying at outlet stores or at online sites such as roadrunnersports.com.

## Question #173: How often should I replace my athletic shoes?

*The short answer:* Replace walking and running shoes every 300 to 500 miles. Other types of shoes should be replaced every three to six months if you use them at least three times a week.

*Every month or so,* place your shoes on a flat surface and inspect them from behind at eye level. If they cave inward or outward quite a bit, it's time for a new pair. The same applies if the treads have worn thin, a fair amount of the stitching is torn, the midsole (the cushioning between the bottom and the body of the shoe) looks compressed, or your joints begin to feel more achy than usual after a workout. Even if your shoes don't look worn on the outside, don't wait more than six months before shopping for a new pair. You may not realize how beat-up your shoes are until you compare them with a fresh pair.

## Question #174: Where should I shop for a treadmill or other home cardio machine?

*The short answer:* You're better off buying from a store that specializes in high-quality exercise equipment than from a department store or, no matter how great the "deal," from a newspaper ad or on eBay.

*There's no downside* to buying dumbbells and barbells at your neighbor's yard sale — there's not much that can go wrong with a hunk of steel. But we strongly advise you to steer clear of department-store treadmills, stationary bikes, and other cardio machines with lots of moving parts; shop instead at a reputable exercise equipment dealer.

Going the specialty-store route will probably cost you a few extra bucks and, in some cases, a lot more than that. But in the end, it's probably worth it. You'll have a better selection of high-quality models and you'll probably get a much better warranty, along with access to someone who knows how to fix the thing if something malfunctions. You may be able to get a bargain by watching for sales and by asking about floor models. Sometimes the salespeople are authorized to give discounts, so it never hurts to ask for one.

Even if you buy from a reputable dealer, do your research. Ask equipment owners for their recommendations. Read reviews from unbiased sources like Consumer Reports. And follow the Golden Rule of equipment purchase: Never buy anything without taking it for a substantial test drive.

## Question #175: What should I look for in a home treadmill?

*The short answer:* At the very least, a treadmill should have a motor, a decent display, and some basic safety features.

*Start with the basic premise* that any treadmill you buy absolutely must have a motorized walking belt. (We explain the pitfalls of motorless models in Question #176.) Look for a machine that doesn't shake or wobble when you use it. We recommend running on it in the store to get a feel for its sturdiness. The display panel should tell you, at the very least, your speed, distance, and calorie burn.

Make sure the machine has side or front rails that you can grasp for balance if necessary. Personally, we like well-designed front rails better. If the side rails extend too far back, you wind up smacking your hands and elbows on them when you swing your arms.

Another key feature is an emergency stop button you can press if you get into trouble. More sophisticated machines have an automatic stop feature that consists of a magnet attached to a cord. The magnet attaches to the display panel, and you clip the cord to your clothing. If you stumble or fall, the magnet breaks its connection with the machine and stops the belt instantly. If you have children or pets or live with someone who acts like a child or a pet, consider paying extra for a model that requires a secret code to start it up.

A decent treadmill will run you at least $1,000. You can spend up to $8,000 for models with fancier features, including extra-wide walking belts, preprogrammed workouts, and displays that give heart-rate feedback and speed-to-pace comparisons. (See Question #138 for definitions of speed and pace.) You certainly don't need to spend top dollar, but we recommend you shop around and test several models before forking over your credit card. Models change all the time, so we can't recommend specific machines, but good manufacturers include True, Precor, Cybex, and TechnoGym.

## Question #176: What's the deal with those motorless treadmills?

*The short answer:* Most of them are flimsier than the premise of a Jackie Chan movie. We've tried dozens of nonmotorized treadmills and have yet to find one we can recommend.

*Nonmotorized treadmills* are enticing because they cost only a few hundred dollars, compared with the $1,000 or more that you have to shell out for a treadmill with a motor. But even at lower prices, the nonmotorized models don't deliver their money's worth.

Motorless treadmills require you to push the walking belt along with your feet. It's nearly impossible to get the belt moving unless you set the machine at an incline, and if you weigh less than 150 pounds, the incline will probably have to be extreme. Beginners who lack leg strength may have to set the machine at such a great incline just to keep the belt moving that they'll tire out after just a few minutes.

At faster walking speeds, nonmotorized belts tend to catch and stick at irregular intervals, causing you to stutter-step along. Forget about taking more than a few running steps on them; it's just too uncomfortable and too hard on your ankle, knee, and hip joints. Plus, there's always a chance the thing will collapse while you're using it. Since they're typically made with the cheapest metal and plastic components, motorless treadmills — especially the handrails — tend to wobble and shake as you move.

## Question #177: What should I look for in a home stationary cycle?

*The short answer:* The most important feature isn't the high-tech display panel, the shiny chrome frame, or the spiffy built-in heart-rate monitor — it's the seat. This applies to all four types of stationary bikes you can choose from: upright, Spinning, recumbent, and cycles with arm attachments.

*All the bells and whistles* money can buy won't make up for a seat that makes you feel like you're perched atop a sack of lumpy potatoes. Don't assume that a wide, soft seat equates to extra comfort. Some people prefer the cushioning, but for others, the extra surface area just means extra friction, and they prefer hard, narrow seats that are more like road-bike saddles. You just can't know your preference unless you take a lengthy test ride. A seat that's comfy for the first 5 minutes may cause you to squirm around 15 minutes later.

Here's what else to look for when you shop for bikes.

### Upright

Upright bikes are similar to outdoor bikes in that you're sitting upright and you pedal up and down. The more expensive models have a computerized panel that displays your cadence, time, heart rate, calorie burn, and more. To increase or decrease the level of difficulty, you just press a button.

The downside of computerization is that it costs megabucks, as much as $2,000 for a really jazzed-up model. For as little as $200, you can buy a no-frills upright equipped with a primitive analog odometer and a knob you can tighten or loosen to change the tension. If forgoing all the fancy feedback doesn't bore you to tears, these lower-end models are a good bargain and most people get just as good a workout. Quality computerized cycle brands include LifeFitness, Cateye, and Cybex. Solid noncomputerized brands include Precor, BodyGuard, and Monarch.

## Spinning

This relatively new stationary cycle category was invented by Johnny Goldberg, better known as Johnny G, the former ultra-distance cyclist who started the group indoor cycling craze. He felt that traditional upright cycles did a lousy job of mimicking the feel and mechanics of outdoor cycling and developed a stationary bike that comes much closer to the real thing. First used in group classes at gyms, these bikes are now marketed to home exercisers, too.

Spin bikes typically don't sport computers, although some companies now offer attachments that display speed, cadence, heart rate, and other features. They have pedals similar to those on an outdoor racing bike and the pedal crank is set farther behind your leg than on an upright cycle. Although you are essentially sitting upright when you spin, the handlebars are lower, so you have to lean forward, as you would on a road bike.

Prices range from about $300 to about $1,200. Quality brands include Star Trac, Reebok, and LeMond.

## Recumbent

Recumbent cycles have a bucket seat that puts you in a slightly reclined position, pedaling out in front of you rather than up and down. Because they provide back support, these bikes are ideal for anyone who has lower back problems, but since your knee moves in toward your chest when you pedal, they're probably not a good choice for someone who's significantly overweight or pregnant.

The recumbents we think are worth recommending are computerized, which means they're on the pricey side — between $1,500 and $2,500. The brands we like are LifeFitness, Cybex, and Precor.

### Cycles with Arm Attachments

Machines such as the Airdyne and CyclePlus have rowing arm attachments that you can push and pull with your arms as you pedal with your legs. Some people consider this feature an advantage. Others find it distracting to work their upper and lower body at the same time.

You'll get a better workout from bikes like the CyclePlus, which have "independent action," meaning that you can set a different intensity level for your upper and lower body; the movement of one doesn't affect the other. With this type of bike, your arms have to work harder to power the rowing action without any help from the legs. However, independent-action bikes have a hefty price tag, running about $4,500. You'll pay about $700 for "dependent" models like the Airdyne, which have the arm and leg movement connected. When you pedal, the arms move even if you're not holding on to them.

## Question #178: What are the most important features of a home elliptical trainer?

***The short answer:*** At the very least, the machine should have a stride length of at least 21 inches, a smooth feel, and adjustments for incline and intensity.

***Elliptical machines*** move like a cross between a treadmill and a stationary bike. They took the gym scene by storm in the mid-1990s, and it was only a few years before manufacturers started producing home models. Unfortunately, most home ellipticals don't offer the quality and the proper body mechanics of their gym counterparts. You have to be an in-

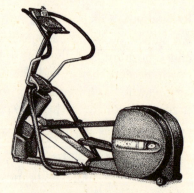

*Elliptical trainers are low impact and easy to use.*

formed buyer indeed to purchase a home elliptical that's worth the metal and plastic it's fashioned from.

When shopping for a home elliptical, make sure it doesn't feel flimsy when you hop aboard. Look for at least a one-year warranty and be sure there's someone who can fix it who lives within driving distance. If you're over 5 feet tall, you need a stride that's at least 21 inches long; otherwise, the motion will feel short and choppy. (The stride length should be listed in the product catalog, but you should also take a test drive to make sure the stride is comfortable for you.) The motion should be smooth, without any kick or catch at either end of the stride. The machine should also have intensity adjustments.

After that, it's all optional bells and whistles, such as preprogrammed workout courses and heart-rate monitor compatibility. Arm attachments typically don't add much in the way of calorie burning or body toning.

As of this writing, good home elliptical trainers are as rare as albino buffalo, although we can recommend home models by Precor, the company that invented the machine. Expect to pay $1,000 to $5,000 for one that's comfortably usable.

## Question #179: Whatever happened to the NordicTrack ski machine?

*The short answer:* The manufacturer went out of business in the late 1990s, but another company bought the name and is currently making home models that are actually a pretty good deal.

*For a few years in the mid-1990s,* NordicTrack ski machines were all the rage, dominating the infomercial airwaves like the fitness version of the George Foreman Grill. Annual sales topped $185 million for these contraptions, which consisted of two arm cords plus wooden skis that slid along a track of rollers. Then, faster than you could say "Lose weight in 20 minutes a day," the NordicTrack vanished. At the end of 1998, the skier's parent company, CML, declared bankruptcy, and suddenly the only way you could purchase a ski machine was on eBay or through your local PennySaver.

What happened? Theories abound. Some believe that the skier was too hard to master — that learning to coordinate the arm and foot movements took more patience and time than most people were willing to invest. Others argue that the skier owed its popularity to the novelty, at the time, of infomercial fitness products, and that like the Aerobic Rider, Ab Roller, Gazelle Glider, and other fitness-equipment fads, it was doomed from the start. But we think the demise of one of the most popular pieces of exercise equipment in history was also in large part due to compromised quality.

When NordicTrack started out, the skis were handcrafted from polished wood; the machine's construction was sturdy, and its action stable and smooth. By the time NordicTrack became an infomercial staple, the company had dumbed it down considerably. Gone were the wooden skis, replaced by cheap metal planks that resembled venetian blinds. The frame wobbled and shook even at slower speeds, and the arm cords and odometers were constantly breaking. Worst of all, there was no customer support. When the machine broke, you couldn't even order the parts to fix it yourself. Despite the massive advertising blitz, the manufacturer couldn't overcome negative word of mouth and consumers moved on to other things, most notably the elliptical trainer.

But that wasn't the end of the NordicTrack. In early 2000 a much larger equipment company, Icon, bought the NordicTrack brand and began reviving it. The company wisely jettisoned the cheaper versions — abandoning the flimsy "club" model that was a big flop with gym-goers — and went back to basics, focusing on high-quality home models with wooden skis. You can now buy the Classic Pro model online at nordictrack.com and at Sears department stores. Although we generally advise against buying cardio equipment online or from department stores (see Question #174), we actually recommend this product. And at about $600, it's a true fitness bargain.

## Question #180: If I'm on a tight budget, what's the best strength-training equipment to buy for my home?

*The short answer:* You don't have to spend a cent to get stronger, but for a truly well-rounded workout, the best values are rubber exercise tubes and steel dumbbells.

*For many exercises* — such as pushups, squats, lunges, and dips — your body weight and gravity provide more than enough resistance to build strength, especially if you're a beginner. To a certain extent, these exercises can be adapted as you get stronger. For example, you can start by doing pushups while standing with your hands pressed against a wall, then graduate to pushups performed on the floor with your knees bent. When that becomes easy, you can do classic pushups, with your legs straight, and when you become a real stud, you can do pushups with your feet on a bed and hands on the floor.

However, not all body-weight exercises are so adaptable, and there are some muscle groups, such as your upper and middle back muscles, that are very difficult to strengthen without some sort of equipment. If you really want to save money, you could scrounge around the house and find items that make good resistance tools because they're easy to grip and because, well, they weigh something. For instance, you can do biceps curls while holding a 16-ounce soup can in each hand. When this becomes easy, do the exercise with a couple of loaded plastic shopping bags. Or, partially fill two bleach bottles with water or sand, adding more sand or water to increase the weight.

However, there's a reason that fitness-equipment stores don't sell jugs of Drano. Equipment that is actually designed for strength training tends to be more versatile and comfortable to use. And it's not even necessarily more expensive. For less than you'd spend on a jar of gourmet jelly, you can buy a set of rubber exercise bands (flat strips of rubber that resemble oversized linguine noodles) or tubes (which resemble giant strands of spaghetti with handles attached). Both varieties cost $6 to $12 apiece and come in several thicknesses.

If you prefer the feel of cold, hard steel and like knowing exactly how much weight you're lifting — which makes it easier to track your progress — the best low-budget option is a set of steel dumbbells. You can buy five pairs — 5, 8, 10, 12, and 15 pounds — for between $50 and $200, depending on the quality and the area of the country you live in. Weight benches, which will make your dumbbells vastly more versatile, start at about $100.

## Question #181: How effective is home equipment like the Soloflex or Total Gym?

*The short answer:* Most of these contraptions can tone and strengthen muscles just fine, as long as you have the patience to assemble them and make the necessary adjustments between exercises. But don't expect to lose 27 pounds of fat in six weeks, as some of the ads promise.

*We can think of a lot worse* fitness purchases than home strength-training machines like the Soloflex, Bowflex, and Total Gym (for instance, the ab belts described in Question #182). You may not be transformed into one of the hunky studmuffins who sell these gizmos on late-night TV, but if you use enough resistance to fatigue your muscles within 8 to 12 repetitions, you should get the same results you would with weight machines or free weights.

These contraptions — basically large frames with a series of cords or large rubber bands attached to metal rods — can certainly save you money and space. Whereas a Soloflex costs about $1,500 and fits into the corner of a room, a high-end multigym can cost upward of ten grand and hog an entire living room.

On the downside, most of these infomercial resistance machines aren't as comfortable or as smooth as machines with weight stacks. And some, like the Bowflex, aren't as safe either. Recently, the company was forced to recall the machines because malfunctioning parts were causing serious injuries to exercisers.

Currently there is a class-action lawsuit pending against Bowflex. Some of these devices give new meaning to the term "assembly required": If you're one of those people stymied by twisting a childproof cap off an aspirin bottle, get ready to spend many frustrating hours trying to piece the darned thing together. Likewise, if it breaks, you're the one who will be stuck trying to determine which thingamajig slipped off which whosiwhatsis. When you buy a machine from a reputable equipment dealer, someone will do the dirty work for you and repairs are just a phone call away.

You also have to learn to adjust the machine between exercises. For example, after you've done a squat you may have to rearrange the various rods and bands in order to do a chest press. All this adds time to your workout and can be so frustrating that it may send you back to watching the infomercials about the contraption rather than actually using it.

Our advice: Test any home strength-training contraption before you buy. Some are so rickety and cheaply made that they'd blow over in a light breeze, and the exercise patterns, seat adjustments, and handle attachments may be awkward to use. It's impossible to determine any of this from a commercial or Web site. You can find some of these items at fitness-equipment dealers or As Seen On TV stores.

## Question #182: Can electronic muscle stimulation belts really tone my abs?

*The short answer:* Can zebras fly? Can Keanu Reeves act?

*Don't believe for one moment* that Fast Abs, Ab Energizer, or any other electronic muscle stimulation (EMS) gizmo will firm, shape, slim, or tone your midsection. The claim that you can "build rock-hard abs with no sweat" is malarkey.

EMS devices do have legitimate uses — they're effective physical therapy tools for relaxing muscle spasms. But building muscle by channeling electrical impulses into your body is a fantasy. EMS gadgets stimulate your muscles to contract, but muscle contraction alone won't do the trick. To become stronger and firmer, your muscles must both contract *and* work to overcome a force such as gravity, a weight, or a rubber band. This is why the abdominal exercises we describe in Question #166 are effective. Fast Abs claims to do "all the work for you," but as with anything in life, you just can't get something for nothing.

EMS products have become such a popular infomercial item that the American Council on Exercise, a nonprofit organization known as "America's workout watchdog," commissioned the University of Wisconsin to test one model. After eight weeks, the subjects who underwent electrical stimulation three times a week on several muscle groups experienced no changes in weight, body-fat percentage, or strength. What's more, they reported that using the gizmo was painful and time-consuming. Each session took about 45 minutes, even after weeks of practice — hmm . . . about the same amount of time it would have taken to do a workout.

Not long ago, the outrageous promises of "washboard abs at the touch of a button" finally caught the eye of the government. In a move dubbed Project Absurd, the Federal Trade Commission sued the marketers of three popular abdominal belts for false advertising. One company was fined more than $10 million, a small price to pay considering the company had bilked hundreds of millions from gullible consumers. Some brands have been removed from the market in response to the lawsuits.

The bottom line: You can't buy flat, tight, strong abs for $49.95 plus shipping and handling. Two or three days a week of focused abdominal training, coupled with plenty of aerobic exercise and a sensible eating plan, is the best route to a toned midsection.

## Question #183: My gym has big plastic balls in the stretching area. What are they for?

*The short answer:* Aside from bouncing it around at the beach, you can use a physioball for hundreds of stretching, strengthening, and balance exercises.

*You've probably seen* one of those colorful, oversized plastic balls sitting in your gym's stretching area and wondered, "What the heck am I supposed to do with that?" Often the ball sits in the corner gathering dust because people don't realize what a great exercise tool it is, especially for stretching. For example, arch your back over the top of a physioball for a mild but effective abdominal and lower back stretch, or drape yourself on the ball facedown to stretch out your shoulders, upper back, and lower back.

Although it doesn't weigh more than a few ounces, a physioball also can make your strength-training routine more challenging. To make a pushup tougher, prop your ankles up on the top of a ball as you perform the exercise. Because the ball wobbles, you have to use a lot more muscle power to hold your body in place as you bend and straighten your arms. To make the exercise even harder, try balancing the underside of your toes on the ball. In Question #166, we demonstrate a physioball crunch.

You can also use the ball to replace a weight bench. Lying on your back on the ball as you perform a dumbbell chest press brings the exercise to a whole new level. You have to engage many deep muscles, especially your transverse abdominals, to keep yourself from rolling off the ball. And while you're building up strength, you're also working on your balance and coordination. Use a lighter weight when you do a resistance training exercise with a ball-bench.

Physioballs, also known as stability balls, cost about $30 and are a great device to have at home. The Web site of the American Council on Exercise, acefitness.org, is a good place to learn basic physioball exercises and buy a high-quality ball. You also can purchase balls from Web sites such as spriproducts.com and bodytrends.com. Several brands come with instructional booklets and videos.

## Question #184: What size physioball should I use?

*The short answer:* When you sit on top of a fully pumped-up ball with your knees bent and feet flat on the floor, your thighs should be parallel to the floor.

*Physioballs* not only come in about a dozen colors, like lime green and blueberry, but they also come in different heights. Proper ball height is important for proper positioning and alignment when you do exercises. Arching your back over the top of a ball that's too small, for instance, will exaggerate the stretch and may wind up hurting your back more than helping it. On the other hand, if you do a seated exercise like a shoulder press while sitting on a ball that's too big, you may have to lean forward in order for your feet to touch the floor. This places excess pressure on your neck and spine.

Here's a handy guide for choosing the right ball size for your height.

### Finding a Ball That Fits

| Ball Height (centimeters) | Your Height |
| --- | --- |
| 45 | 5'4" or shorter |
| 55 | 5'5"–5'7" |
| 65 | 5'8"–6' |
| 75 | 6'1" or taller |

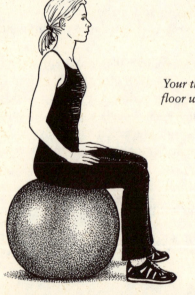

*Your thighs should be parallel to the floor when you sit on top of the ball.*

# Question #185: How accurate are pedometers?

*The short answer:* They vary quite a bit. Many are accurate enough to estimate the number of steps you take, although research shows pedometers tend to be less accurate for clocking mileage and even less accurate for counting calories burned.

*Do you have any idea* how many steps you take in a day? Most of us have no clue, but there's good reason to find out. By some estimates, if we all walked an extra 2,000 steps a day, the vast majority of the U.S. population could avoid the weight gain that has made us the most overweight industrialized nation in the world.

Of course, it would be mighty distracting to go around counting your steps all day ("Wait, was I on 6,458 or 6,469?"). That's where a pedometer — a beeper-sized device that you clip onto your waistband — comes in handy. You measure your average stride length and program it into the pedometer. Inside there's a small pendulum that counts off a step every time you move your hip. For most people, a mile of walking is about 2,000 to 2,500 steps. A sedentary person takes about 5,000 steps a day. (A study on the Amish, by contrast, shows that they take as many as 18,000 steps a day! See Question #4.)

If you're curious to know how you stack up, choose a Japanese brand such as Yamax, suggests David Bassett, Jr., a professor of exercise science at the University of Tennessee, Knoxville, who has researched the accuracy of pedometers. "Japanese pedometers are quite accurate. The ones from China and Taiwan aren't as good." In one study of 13 different models, Bassett found that some pedometers underestimated the number of steps by 25 percent, whereas others overestimated by 45 percent. Five of the 13 were deemed accurate. Another study of 10 models found that most estimated distance to within 10 percent at moderate speeds, but overestimated distance at slower speeds and underestimated it at faster speeds.

Wearing a pedometer can inspire you to become more active. This way, you get credit for every step you take — to your boss's office, to the ATM, around the supermarket, and through the dog park.

## Question #186: Should I hire a personal trainer?

*The short answer:* Personal trainers aren't just for famously fit folks like P. Diddy, Oprah, and Britney. If you don't know a lunge from a leg press, if you're striving for a specific goal, if you're in a rut, or if you haven't picked up a weight since Jack LaLanne was the reigning king of fitness, you're a good candidate for at least a few sessions with a trainer.

*Hiring a trainer* need not be a lifelong commitment. Just three sessions — which will cost you $100 to $500, depending on where you live — can be enough to get you up and running or to breathe new life into a stale routine. A qualified trainer will gently lead you through the basics, ensuring that you don't sit on a machine backward or tear your rotator cuff because you pulled on the wrong lever. With a trainer's help, you can learn to perfect your technique and structure a sound workout program.

As you progress, you may want to stick with training a while longer or even go back for a few tune-up sessions every few months to keep from falling into a rut. Any trainer worth his or her salt can show you a dozen different ways to work your chest, 16 tricks for toning your thighs, and 50 ways to leave your love handles. Besides, having an appointment that you *pay* for and a specific time you're required to show up for exercise can be invaluable.

Personal training is also helpful for anyone who's striving to achieve a goal, such as preparing for a backpacking trip or firming up for your wedding. Many trainers have specialties, such as yoga or fitness over 50, so choose one with expertise and experience in designing programs to meet goals such as yours. As we explain in question #187, make sure your trainer has the proper credentials.

## Question #187: What qualifications should my personal trainer have?

*The short answer:* Look for the same attributes you'd seek in any employee: education, experience, and a personal style that meshes with yours.

A *personal trainer* can give you the inspiration and training advice that you need to achieve your goals, but a trainer can also be a big waste of money — or worse, a source of pain and aggravation — if you end up with the wrong one. Some people shrink from asking about a trainer's credentials, assuming that anyone whose business card says "Personal Trainer" knows more about exercise than they do. But as in any field, trainers run the gamut from highly qualified to total quack. Since you're probably paying at least $35 per session, if not quite a bit more, and you're trusting this person with no less than your body, it makes sense to choose someone who knows his annular ligament from his elbow. On the other hand, don't be unduly impressed by trainers who throw around terms like annular ligament. A command of anatomical jargon does not guarantee competence as a trainer. Neither, by the way, does a great body.

At an absolute minimum, your trainer should hold a current certification from one of the major professional fitness organizations that we describe in Question #188. This at least assures you that he or she is committed enough to have learned training basics and to keep up with the times. (To keep certifications current, trainers must take a certain number of continuing-education classes every year.) It's even better if, in addition to the certification, the trainer has earned a bachelor's or master's degree in a fitness-related field such as physical education or exercise physiology (the study of human muscular, skeletal, circulatory, and nervous systems and how they respond to exercise).

We like private personal trainers who have had at least two years' experience in a health club. In this amount of time, they're generally able to pick up the key tricks of the trade, things that they can learn only from being around other trainers and experimenting with clients. Trainers with in-depth experience can probably teach you at least 15 versions of the squat and know just the right exercise to firm up that spot just below your armpit. They'll also have the skills to motivate you when you're feeling lazy, the networking capabilities to get you a deal on a home treadmill, the good sense to carry liability insurance, and the know-how to implement some simple measurements that can help gauge your progress.

Of course, we're assuming that these trainers paid attention during their health-club tenure. We've come across plenty who were so busy watching a basketball game on the gym's TV that they failed to notice their clients performing repetitions too quickly and with terrible form. We wondered what else they missed during their training careers.

Ideally, your trainer should not only get you to push out an extra repetition on the leg-extension machine, but he or she should also teach you some independence. On the days when you work out on your own, you shouldn't stand there puzzled over how to adjust the seat on that leg extension or which exercise to do next. Your trainer should teach you routines that you can do on your own and clue you in as to why it's not okay to squat until your butt touches the floor. For all you're paying, you should come away with a working knowledge of working out.

That said, even a trainer who has plenty of education, experience, and dedication still won't get you to show up for a 5:30 A.M. session if the two of you aren't on the same wavelength. Ask yourself what type of personal style you respond to: the drill-sergeant-in-*Full-Metal-Jacket* approach or the shrink-in-*The-Prince-of-Tides* approach? Try to get a recommendation from someone you trust so you can get a sense of the trainer's style before you shell out any money.

If you do all of your homework and still end up with a trainer who intimidates you, annoys you, or just isn't getting you results, don't be afraid to go elsewhere. It may take some trial and error before you find the trainer who suits you.

## Question #188: Which certifications should my trainer have?

*The short answer:* At the very least, your trainer should have a personal training certification from the American College of Sports Medicine, the American Council on Exercise, the National Academy of Sports Medicine, or the National Strength and Conditioning Association.

*Certification* is the absolute minimum requirement for a personal trainer. Getting a decent certification requires passing a test that covers anatomy, workout design, safe exercise technique, and other important topics. However, there are more than 360 certifications offered, and they are not all created equal. Some can be "earned" through the Internet and require little more than 90 bucks and your e-mail address. One online certification test provides an answer key and lets you take the exam over and over until you pass it.

Currently there are four certifying organizations generally considered by the legitimate exercise community to fit the bill: the American College of Sports Medicine (ACSM), the American Council on Exercise (ACE), the National Academy of Sports Medicine (NASM), and the National Strength and Conditioning Association (NSCA). Their tests and study materials are designed by top fitness professionals, from respected trainers to Ph.D. researchers, and cover the type of information that trainers need to know in order to provide a good — and safe — workout. These are also the only four organizations that have either gained, or are in the process of filing for, an accreditation similar to the type of accreditation that respected academic institutions and national exams like the SAT and MCAT have earned.

But even within these organizations there are different levels of certification, some more demanding than others and some more appropriate for personal trainers. For instance, the ACSM Health Fitness Instructor certification, geared toward personal trainers, requires passing a stringent written evaluation as well as a challenging practical exam. The trainer must demonstrate technical skills on everything from performing a submaximal bike test to proper spotting technique for the squat. Most people take a three- to five-day workshop in order to pass it. On the other hand, the ACSM Exercise Leadership certification is aimed at instructors of group classes such as step aerobics and kickboxing. The leadership exam doesn't require as much technical knowledge as the health-fitness instructor test, but it does require a thorough understanding of topics like how to select music for a warm-up and how to modify a step move for someone who has creaky knees.

The ACE Personal Trainer and Certified Exercise Specialist certifications are designed for trainers, whereas the organization's Group Fitness Instructor and Lifestyle Weight Management certification require a lower level of knowledge. The personal-trainer exam is fairly basic, while the exercise-specialist test requires more advanced knowledge, such as how to modify a workout for someone who has high blood pressure. The trainer exam now includes a "practical simulation" section, consisting of a series of questions designed to determine a trainer's response to typical situations, such as choosing exercises for a client who has bad knees.

The NASM has two levels of certification: the Certified Professional Trainer and the Performance Enhancement Specialist. The CPT certification is geared toward fitness professionals planning to work in a health club with clients who have general fitness goals. The PES certification is designed for those who plan to work with athletes in an athletic-training environment such as a professional team, college, or clinic.

The NSCA offers two excellent certifications for personal trainers: Certified Strength Conditioning Specialist and Certified Personal Trainer. The CSCS is an advanced certification requiring sophisticated knowledge of weight-training technique. The CPT is a lot more basic but a good entry-level credential. Both certifications require passing a written and practical video exam. For example, candidates watch a video of someone doing a lunge and then must answer questions about technique, muscle usage, and alternative exercises. The NSCA exams are widely considered to be the most thorough when it comes to testing weight-training knowledge and form.

Other certifications worth considering are those developed by local colleges and universities. In many cases, these may be earned after a couple of semesters of classes, and they generally require in-depth knowledge and hands-on experience. However, even if a trainer has one of these certifications, he or she should also have one of the "Big Four" mentioned above.

Consumers beware: Just because a trainer has earned a certification doesn't necessarily mean the credential is current. Some trainers don't bother to renew their certifications on a regular basis, which means they aren't really certified. Worse, some trainers lie about having a certification in the first place. The ACSM, ACE, NASM, and NSCA all have databases of their certified trainers, so you can call to verify your trainer's resume — ACSM: (317) 637-9200; ACE: (800) 825-3636; NASM: (800) 460 6276; NSCA: (800) 815-6826. You can find local certified trainers through these organizations' Web sites at ascm.org, acefitness.org, nasm.org, and nsca-lift.org.

Most certifications expire after one or two years unless the trainer earns continuing education credits, either by attending conferences, taking monthly quizzes or workshops, participating in research projects, or performing community service in a fitness center. This requirement is great for the consumer: You want your trainer to keep up on fitness trends, training techniques, and research, and this system provides incentive for trainers to do so.

## Question #189: How do I know if my group-exercise instructor is any good?

*The short answer:* Does the instructor offer encouragement, ask for feedback, and clue you in on different ways to do each move? Does she face the class rather than operate in her own little world? If you answer yes to these questions, chances are the teacher knows her stuff, although you should still inquire about her credentials.

*The group-workout world* is pretty diverse. The skills required of a great strip aerobics instructor are vastly different from those of, say, a meditative yoga teacher. To further complicate matters, certification requirements aren't as uniformly agreed upon as they are for personal trainers. It's a real challenge for consumers to evaluate whether a group instructor has the chops to lead an exercise class.

Still, all good instructors have the same basic traits: experience, education, empathy, and a teaching style that keeps students from tripping over their feet, collapsing from exhaustion, or quitting out of boredom. Some of this is a matter of personal preference, of course. Certain exercisers respond best to instructors with a cheerleader flair while others prefer a more Marine-like approach. But it's a wise idea to find out whether an instructor, inspiring as she may be, knows her rectus abdominis from her levator scapula.

If you're uncomfortable asking the instructor herself, check with the club to see if your teacher is certified by a national professional organization, such as the American Council on Exercise, that specifically tests for group-class acumen rather than personal-training skills. However, for instructors of yoga, Spinning, Pilates, and other so-called specialty classes, a mainstream certification may not apply. The mainstream creds can be a real plus, but these classes should be taught by a specialist who has earned credentials specific to that field.

Most group-class instructors don't hold degrees in fields such exercise physiology or biomechanics, but often have extensive backgrounds in dance, gymnastics, or sports. This can be good or bad. Some instructors are such theater divas that they don't know how to tone it down for the masses. They think that folding themselves in half like a lawn chair comes naturally to most people and teach moves that are often beyond the capabilities of mere mortals. On the other hand, a dance background can mean a solid understanding of how the body can and can't move.

In the end, though, rely on your own instincts. If an instructor doesn't float your boat, even if she has a cult following, try another class.

**Question #190: How can I get a good deal on a health-club membership?**

*The short answer:* The best strategy is to *ask* for a good deal.

*Oftentimes health club* salespeople are authorized to give discounts, waive initiation fees, tack on free extra months of membership, or give away free training sessions. But they don't unless they have to. Most club salespeople work on commission, so it's in their best interest to make the most expensive sale possible. At the same time, making a discounted sale is better than making no sale at all.

You may also score a better deal if you go in with a friend or family member. Some clubs offer discounted rates when two or more people join together (but again, you may have to specifically ask for this). If you work for a corporation, even if it isn't a giant conglomerate, check to see if your company has negotiated a discount, which may be as much as 50 percent. If your company hasn't already done this, you may be able to get an account set up through your human resources or corporate services department.

Also be on the lookout for sales, which tend to happen in the summer, when the gym business is slower, or during January, when clubs try to lasso in all of the New Year's resolution types. You can also try going in on the last day of the month, when salespeople are trying to make their quotas. This is also the best time to ask for discounts.

Of course, you can try a reverse-psychology tactic like walking out and coming back the next day. Just remember that these guys and gals have seen it all. Your return may nudge them into giving you a lower price, but it's just as likely to send a signal that you want the membership badly enough to come back a second time. But hey, it costs nothing but a little extra time to try.

Once you've negotiated your membership rate, read all contracts carefully before signing them. You may find that that deal you negotiated isn't such a steal after all if you wind up having to pay locker fees, towel fees, group-class fees, and parking fees. Don't sign up for more than one year, no matter how great the deal is, and read the cancellation and membership clauses thoroughly. Some of them are harsher and more ironclad than a jail sentence. Many big club chains tack on huge penalties if you try to wiggle out of your membership or are even a day late with your fees.

# How Exercise Affects Your Health: Back Pain, Osteoporosis, Depression, and More

You don't need a marketing degree to figure out why "Flat Abs in 4 Weeks!" and "The Quick Weight-Loss Solution!" are the type of slogans used to sell exercise programs and equipment. Naturally, most people work out because they want to look slimmer and firmer as quickly as possible, so you're not going to see many infomercial hosts saying things like, "Reduce your diabetes risk!" or "Stave off Syndrome X!"

Yet exercise has benefits that extend way beyond toned abs and sculpted thighs. More and more, researchers are discovering that exercise is as effective as — if not more effective than — medication to help fight or reduce your risk of developing many diseases and health conditions. In this section, we cover how exercise affects a whole host of conditions, from back pain to diabetes to cancer to depression. We also cover the reverse: how your health affects your workouts. For instance, is it okay to exercise when you have a cold? When you have lower back pain? When you haven't slept much?

Chances are, looking good will always be the number one reason that most people swim, bike, hike, run, step, and lift. But for some of us, feeling good and staying healthy are becoming increasingly more important.

## Question #191: Is it okay to exercise when I have a cold?

*The short answer:* Yes, as long as you don't have a fever and don't overdo it.

*If you have a run-of-the-mill case* of the sniffles and aren't feeling too rundown, it's okay to get your heart rate up a bit and break a mild sweat, doctors say. But use common sense and listen to your body. The day you wake up with a runny nose, watery eyes, and scratchy throat is not the day to take a firefighter boot camp class. And if you have a fever, doctors say, exercise is verboten. A fever signals that your immune system is fighting the infection aggressively, and that's not a process you want to interfere with.

If you're feeling well enough to work out, cut your usual time and intensity by about half. Also, make sure you drink more fluid than usual, since you'll already be fighting dehydration from being sick. Oh, and if you're coughing up phlegm and your nose is dripping like a leaky faucet, do your fellow exercisers a favor and keep yourself and your germs away from the gym. A few days away from the treadmill won't cause your fitness to evaporate and may be exactly what your body needs to recover.

If you're unsure whether you're healthy enough to work out, consult your doctor.

## Question #192: Do exercisers get sick less often than people who don't work out?

*The short answer:* Yes. Regular, moderate workouts make you less susceptible to colds and infections.

*The evidence is compelling:* In three studies that tracked a total of 160 unfit women, including some who were elderly and others who were overweight, those who started walking briskly five days a week for 45 minutes logged half the number of sick days over a 12- to 15-week period as the women who didn't exercise. Other studies have suggested that 30 minutes of moderate exercise on most days of the week offers immune-system benefits, and several work-site studies have found that employees who regularly use the company gym use a lot fewer sick days than employees who don't work out.

How exactly does breaking a sweat boost immunity? When

your body is at rest, most of your immune cells — the ones pro-grammed to fight infection — hibernate in certain places, such as your lymph nodes, spleen, and bone marrow. But when you work out, research shows, "a lot of these cells come pouring out of those depots and start circulating around," says exercise and im-munity expert David Nieman, Ph.D., director of the human per-formance laboratory at Appalachian State University in Boone, North Carolina. He likens this activity to cops pouring out of the station house and into the streets to catch up with the crooks. About three hours after a workout, the immune cells go back into hiding, but stimulating your immune system day after day seems to give you more consistent protection against viruses.

## Question #193: Am I more likely to get sick after a killer workout than a more moderate one?

*The short answer:* Yes, very long, hard workouts can suppress the immune system in a big way, leaving you more susceptible to in-fections for up to three days.

*It's called the "open window" theory:* In the period from three hours to 72 hours after strenuous endurance exercise, dramatic changes in your immune system, including increased levels of stress hormones, leave you open to infection. Recent studies on athletic competitions have made strides toward proving this the-ory. For instance, researchers monitored 100 competitors in the Western States, a grueling 100-mile running race in the Sierra Nevada mountains that took participants about 27 hours to com-plete. Blood and saliva samples taken before, during, and after the event indicated the racers' immune systems had been radically suppressed. In the two weeks following the event, a whopping 25 percent of the runners reported upper-respiratory-tract infections. The runners who had the lowest levels of a certain throat-protect-ing antibody were the most likely to get sick.

Another study compared competitors in the L.A. marathon with runners who trained for the race but, for various reasons, did not participate in the event. In the two weeks following the marathon, 13 percent of the racers got sick, compared with 2 percent of the runners who didn't race. In other words, those who raced were six times more likely to come down with a cold.

Do you have to go marathon distance before your immune system weakens? Probably not, but it takes about 90 minutes of consecutive, high-intensity exercise to significantly depress immune function. Researchers have measured athletes in training and in competition and have found the largest immune changes during races.

Even if long, strenuous workouts take a toll on your immune system, this doesn't mean you're doomed to get sick after your next marathon or bike race. Research suggests that consuming 60 grams of carbohydrates — such as a liter of Gatorade — for every hour of strenuous exercise can counteract the depressed immune function that's so common after endurance events. Carbohydrates keep your blood sugar high, which seems to diminish the amount of stress hormones released during prolonged, intense exercise. "It works amazingly well," says David Nieman, of Appalachian State University, who has tested the effects of several substances, including carbohydrates, on the immune systems of athletes.

## Question #194: Is there anything I can do for an attack of back pain?

*The short answer:* Yes, there are plenty of pain-relief remedies you can try, such as applying heat or ice, taking anti-inflammatory medication, getting a gentle massage, and having your spine manipulated by a back-pain specialist.

*Have you ever* bent over to pick up a fork and felt like you'd just had a knife stuck in your back? At some point, nearly 80 percent of adult Americans experience lower back pain and nearly 60 percent of lower back pain sufferers experience chronic pain. Exercise sometimes can be the cause of lower back pain; at other times, it can also help alleviate such pain. But during the first 48 to 72 hours of a back episode, the best therapy is simply to rest, moving around as little as possible, says Evan Johnson, P.T., advanced clinical physical therapy coordinator for the New York Presbyterian Spine Center. You can also apply ice for up to 15 minutes at a time during this crucial period, although never place it directly in contact with your skin.

While your back is in pain, make sure you avoid anything that makes it feel worse. "Sitting is particularly hard on the spine," Johnson says, because all of your lower spine muscles that aren't in spasm are relaxed and therefore unable to provide support or shock absorption to the spine. You may find some relief from back-support pillows or posture straps, girdle-like contraptions that compress the spine and force you into a more upright posture than normal. When you do sit or stand, take extra care to avoid slouching, which can throw off your spinal alignment and make matters worse.

For the first three days of back pain, apply ice, not heat (heat increases inflammation). It can penetrate deep enough below the surface muscles to dull the pain, providing temporary relief. Ice also helps by controlling swelling and inflammation.

Research has also shown that anti-inflammatories, gentle massage, and manual manipulation of the spine by a physical therapist, osteopath, or chiropractor can be effective back-pain relievers. But don't bother with ultrasound or electrical stimulation, Johnson says. These common treatments may give you an hour or two of relief, but that's usually about it.

After 72 hours of back pain, Johnson says, "you're probably as inflamed as you're going to get," so from that point on, some light movement can help relax the discomfort. Johnson recommends walking, swimming, and careful stretching to loosen up tight muscles and increase blood flow to the lower back muscles. The exercises in Question #195 may also help.

If you've done everything right and are still in agony after a few days, get yourself to a doctor. One reason so many people have lifelong back pain is because they were diagnosed incorrectly — or not diagnosed at all. "Most low back pain clears up on its own within six weeks, and once the immediate episode is over, there's a tendency to put it out of your mind until the next time," Johnson says. By going to a doctor who specializes in treating back pain, you can get to the root of the problem — maybe you tried lifting a stack of Harry Potter novels or hacked up too many clods of dirt on the fairway — and resolve it rather than just treating the symptoms.

## Question #195: What are the best exercises I can do to ease lower back pain?

*The short answer:* If you're unable to stand up straight or feel like your spine has been run over by a truck, exercise may not help you — and may make matters worse. But if you're experiencing some general stiffness or achiness or have back pain on a consistent basis, stretching and strengthening exercises may offer some relief.

*"The best way* to eliminate or at least decrease back pain is to increase your hip, thigh, and spinal flexibility and strength," says physical therapist Evan Johnson of the New York Presbyterian Spine Center at Columbia Presbyterian Medical Center in New York City. Below are four exercises that Johnson recommends. Do one to three sets of each exercise two or three times a week. You should start to feel better immediately and should feel substantial relief within one month. If you don't feel any better or find these exercises painful, check with your doctor.

### Hamstring Stretch

This stretch eases the tug of your hamstring muscles on your hips, enabling your spine to relax and move toward a more ideal posture.

Lie on your back with your knees bent and your feet flat on the floor, hip width apart. Lift your leg and grasp your calf with both hands, straighten your knees as much as you comfortably can, and gently pull your leg toward you until you feel a gentle tug through the back of your thigh. Hold for 30 seconds, the recommended length of time for stretching an injured muscle, then re-

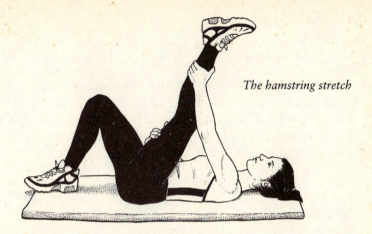

*The hamstring stretch*

peat with your other leg. If you don't have the flexibility to reach your calf, loop a towel around your calf and hold on to the ends.

## Pretzel Stretch

This stretch loosens up the hips, especially the outer hips, which helps relax and align your lower back.

Lie on your back with your left knee bent, foot flat on the floor, and your right ankle resting across the top of your left thigh. Now lift your legs so that your left thigh is perpendicular to the floor. Clasp your hands around your left thigh and gently pull it back toward you. Hold for 30 seconds and repeat on the other side.

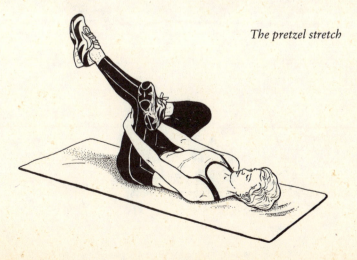

*The pretzel stretch*

## The Anchor

This exercise uses all of your abdominal muscles, including the deepest ones that attach to the muscles of the lower spine.

A. Lie on your back with your left knee bent, foot on the floor. Lift your right leg up off the floor, and bend your knee so that the lower leg is parallel to the floor and the upper leg is directly in line with your hip. Flex your heel. Raise your arms up over your chest and clasp your fingers together.

B. Slowly lower your heel toward the floor and your arms back and behind your head. Keep your abs pulled inward. Don't let your lower back pop off the floor. This becomes harder as your heel and hands move closer to the floor. When your heel has almost touched the floor, slowly return your arms and leg to the starting position. Do three reps for each side.

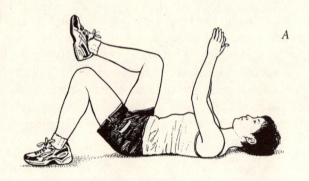

A

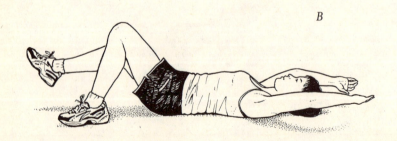

B

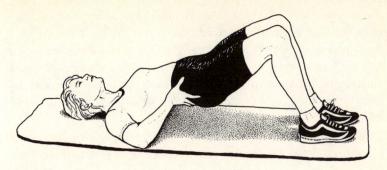

### Bridging

This exercise works the deepest abdominal muscles.

A. Lie on your back with your knees bent and feet flat on the floor about hip width apart. Rest your arms wherever they're most comfortable. Gently press your back down and pull your abdominals toward your spine. Don't tilt your head up and back.

B. Press your feet downward, pull your abs inward and tuck your pelvis so that you gently curl your entire back, from your butt to your shoulder blades, off the floor. Hold this position for five slow counts and slowly roll back down to the starting position.

### Question #196: If I have lower back problems, which strength-training exercises should I avoid?

*The short answer:* It's a simple rule — any exercise that bothers your back! Exercises that traditionally are troublemakers include twisting movements, overhead pressing exercises, and exercises in which you're likely to overarch your back. But just about any exercise can wrench your back if you use poor technique.

*The lower back* is a notoriously delicate area, comprising dozens of tiny, intricate muscles and ligaments that are easily pulled or strained. That's why more than 80 percent of us experience pain in the last five vertebrae of our spine at some time or another. Since your lower back is involved in virtually every movement you do, whether this region is actually moving or whether it's simply tightening up to stabilize your body as some other part moves, it finds plenty of opportunity to get into trouble. Lower back pain can also be caused by a wearing away of the disks that create cushioning between your vertebrae; when this cushy cartilage disintegrates, with age or extensive use, you're left with bone grinding against bone — ouch.

While exercise is often the key to preventing or curing back pain, if you're not careful, strength training can exacerbate lower back troubles. When you perform pressing movements — whether it's an overhead shoulder press, a bench press, or a even a leg press — don't try to set any personal weight records. You'll only end up twisting or arching your back as a sort of a cheat to lift the extra poundage. Be sure to tighten your abdominals to create additional stability and support for your lower back.

In some cases, arching your back is actually a legitimate part of the exercise. When you perform these moves, such as the back hyperextension, a back raise done on the floor or on a special bench, move into the arch carefully and don't force yourself past your natural arch. The same advice applies to yoga positions that call for you to lie on your stomach and lift your chest, legs, or both off the floor. You may even want to forgo all back-arching exercises. Some people just aren't built for them, and they may be the proverbial straw that breaks the camel's back.

Take the same slow and cautious approach to any movement that involves twisting. If you build up too much momentum, you may stress your back muscles faster than you can stop the movement. Keeping your abs pulled in will help stabilize and protect your lower back.

We've just described the exercises that are in the pain-in-the-back hall of fame. However, persistently bad form on just about any exercise can send your back into a tizzy. Leaning backward during a heavy biceps curl, setting your seat too high or low, even something as innocent as bending over the wrong way to pick up a weight can do you in. Some lifting mistakes may not take you down immediately but may instead haunt you over time. We recommend getting professional instruction whenever you add a new exercise to your repertoire. It may save you a few days of applying ice packs and popping painkillers.

Even if you use stellar form and avoid those pressing, arching, and twisting moves, there still may be some exercises you should simply avoid. You know how you meet someone at a party and you just don't hit it off no matter how hard you try? Well, the same is true of some exercises and certain people. When you run into a move that causes your lower back to ping, even if you're doing everything right, it's best to agree to disagree with it and part company forever.

## Question #197: My knees make a clicking sound when I do certain exercises. What's causing this, and should I worry?

*The short answer:* Snapping and popping sounds are typically caused by ligaments or tendons moving roughly over the kneecap, a condition called *crepitis*. Crepitis can sometimes be a precursor to chronic knee problems such as torn cartilage, so if your knees are also chronically swollen, red, and painful, see a doctor immediately.

*A normal, healthy kneecap* sits in a little groove between your upper and lower leg bones, and when you bend and straighten your knee, it moves straight up and down along this track. But when your thigh muscles, ligaments, and tendons are tight, they can pull your kneecap slightly to the outside. As a result, every time you move your knee it sounds like a pencil being snapped in half. This sound is most likely caused by the grinding of the thighbone and kneecap as it tries to form new, misaligned grooves.

Although clicky knees aren't always painful, they are a sign of imbalances and abnormal wear and tear. Regular stretching and strengthening of the hamstrings, quadriceps, and outer thighs will probably reduce the noise, as well as your chances of injury. The way that your foot hits the ground affects the movement of your knee, so wear shoes that have good heel support and that keep your foot from rolling excessively inward or outward. Over-the-counter arch supports or custom-made orthotics also can help keep your entire leg, from your arch to your hip, in proper alignment.

## Question #198: Is it okay to feel sore after a workout?

*The short answer:* Yes, as long as you're not so sore that combing your hair hurts and as long as you're not sore on a regular basis.

*When we say "muscle soreness,"* we're talking about a dull, general achiness — not the sharp, specific pain you feel when you've damaged a muscle, tendon, or ligament. Sharp pain is not normal, and if it persists for more than a few days, we recommend a trip to a medical professional.

Muscle soreness comes in two varieties. The kind you feel during or immediately after a killer workout is the result of lactic acid (defined in Question #126) flooding into your muscles. It's very intense and usually a signal that you're reaching your limits and need to stop. Most people don't have the ability to push through this kind of pain, nor do they have any reason to, although you often see lactic acid–induced expressions of agony on Olympic runners sprinting across the finish line. This kind of soreness usually subsides within 15 minutes of a workout, as the lactic acid gets flushed out of your muscles.

The type of muscle soreness you feel one or two days after a particularly hard workout is called delayed onset muscle soreness, or, if you like exercise acronyms, DOMS. It happens when microscopic tears in your muscle fibers — tears that are the normal result of a hard cardio or strength workout — fill up with blood from broken vessels along with the various waste products created by your body when you exercise really hard.

It's okay to feel DOMS a couple of times a month. In fact, you should expect to feel this kind of soreness for a few days after starting an exercise program or after a layoff of a week or two. But most people adapt to exercise, even hard exercise, in a period of a few weeks and don't experience DOMS all that often. If you're regularly waking up so sore that you can barely walk down a flight of stairs, you need to cut back on the number of intense workouts you do.

When you experience DOMS, ease up for a day or two or take a few days off to let your body recoup. Some people find that a light cardio workout the day after a heavy one helps alleviate soreness, but if you're really sore after a hard weight-training session, don't lift again until you're over the soreness, and when you do lift, keep it on the light side.

If you're feeling completely wrecked after an especially hard workout or competition, consider getting a massage, a remedy that exercise experts and athletes, including us, swear by, despite scant evidence that massage reduces muscle soreness.

## Question #199: What fitness activity has the highest injury rate?

*The short answer:* It won't come as a shock to anyone that tackle football has a higher percentage of traumatic injuries than any other sport, racking up 40 injuries for every 1,000 hours of play. But who'd have guessed badminton has the highest rate of overuse injuries? Running, not surprisingly, is the endurance activity with the highest injury rate.

*About 17 percent* of the 20 million or so annual athletic injuries — from broken legs due to snowboarding to dislocated shoulders from doing a face plant off a mountain bike — require a trip to the emergency room, according to Sports Data, Inc., an organization that tracks trends in sports and fitness activities. But most injuries — the typical sprains, strains, and bruises — just keep participants sidelined for days or weeks.

Most fitness-related injuries are the result of overuse rather than a single catastrophe. When an athlete's body simply can't stand up to the constant demands of exercise, eventually the knees go, the ankles give out, or the lower back acts up. This happens frequently to runners. As a direct result of pounding the pavement, as many as 65 percent of recreational runners a year wind up limping, hobbling, or worse. The average runner misses 5 to 10 percent of workouts due to injury. In contrast, only about 21 percent of walkers and 7 percent of people who train with weights get hurt each year.

Believe it or not, badminton players have the highest rate of overuse injuries for any sport. About 85 percent of them experience an injury each year, mainly to the Achilles tendon, lower back, elbow, or shoulder. Badminton players also have a high percentage of traumatic eye injuries.

Although some injuries can't be prevented — getting whacked in the head by a hockey puck, for instance — wearing proper equipment can help reduce your chances of getting seriously hurt by those one-in-a-million mishaps. To diminish your risk of overuse injuries, choose high-quality gear, including athletic shoes that fit; keep your muscles and joints strong and flexible; and avoid too many consecutive days of high-intensity exercise.

## Question #200: Can cycling make a man impotent?

*The short answer:* Perhaps. Heavier men and men who ride more than 10 hours a week are most likely to experience cycling-related impotence, but specially designed seats may help rectify the problem.

*If you're male* and spend a long time in the saddle, cycling may be hazardous to your sex life. In fact, the problem seems to be the saddle itself. On most bicycles, the rider presses his weight forward, compromising or cutting off completely the blood supply to the cavernosal artery, which supplies blood to the penis. Research shows that it takes just 11 percent of body weight to compress this artery. If it is frequently compressed over a long period of time — well, no blood flow, no erection. A study of more than 500 men found that nearly 4 percent of them suffered from impotence. By comparison, only 1 percent of the non-cyclists studied were afflicted.

The National Institute for Occupational Safety and Health (NIOSH) even looked into this issue after learning that police officers on bicycle duty were complaining of genital numbness and erectile dysfunction. In a study of bike cops and non-riders, NIOSH tested the duration of nighttime erection, a strong indicator of overall sexual health. The upshot: The non-cyclists experienced erection during 43 percent of their sleep cycle, compared with only 27 percent for the bike cops. Among the bike cops — who averaged 5.4 hours per day in the saddle — a whopping 93 percent reported experiencing groin numbness on occasion.

Research like this has caused bike manufactures to rethink seat design. For instance, the makers of Specialized bikes teamed up with a physician to create the Body Geometry Seat, a Y-shaped saddle with the rear portion removed to reduce pressure on critical arteries. The company seems to have the right idea. A number of studies have found that Body Geometry and other specially designed saddles can offer complete or partial relief to male cyclists with symptoms ranging from groin numbness to impotence. (There are also saddles designed specially for women, who may also be susceptible to genital numbness after long hours spent in the saddle.)

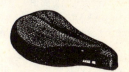

*A specialized bike seat helps reduce numbness.*

Besides switching to a new bike seat, doctors recommend pointing your saddle a few degrees downward to avoid compression of key areas. To prevent excessive forward body lean, set your seat height so that your knee is slightly bent at the bottom of the pedal stroke. Stand in the pedals every ten minutes or so, even while riding a stationary bike, to restore blood flow to the crotch and penis. When riding over bumpy terrain, stand up, bend your knees slightly, and use your legs rather than your crotch as shock absorbers. Switching to a recumbent cycle, the kind where you sit in a bucket seat and pedal out in front of you, will also help, but this style of bike comes with its own risks, namely ridicule from serious cyclists who consider it ultra-dorky.

If you are a cyclist who has experienced chronic numbness, excessive genital shrinkage, pain in the groin, or impotence, see your urologist.

## Question #201: Will I sleep better if I exercise?

*The short answer:* You might sleep a bit longer than usual after a workout, but research suggests you probably won't fall asleep more quickly or sleep more soundly.

*Conventional wisdom* has it that exercise sends you into a deeper, longer slumber, and there's some research to back that up. The problem: The research has generally relied on personal reports. When scientists actually monitor their subjects' brain-wave patterns or wrist activity (a measure that has been correlated with brain-wave activity), the conventional wisdom hasn't held up. "If you question people, they say they sleep better, but if you look at it objectively, exercise has a very modest effect on sleep," says sleep researcher Shawn Youngstedt, Ph.D., of the University of California, San Diego.

In a review of 38 studies on sleep and exercise, Youngstedt found that aerobic exercise increased total sleep time on average by 10 minutes and had almost no effect on how quickly subjects fell asleep or the number of sleep disturbances they experienced. (Most of the research has looked at aerobic workouts, so it is unknown whether weight training, stretching, or yoga promotes better slumber.) The sleep benefits of a gym visit or a jaunt around the neighborhood seem to be greatest when workouts last longer than one hour.

It's not clear whether regular exercisers sleep longer or more soundly than couch potatoes, since most sleep studies have considered how a single session of exercise affects sleep. In surveys, avid exercisers do report sleeping better than people who don't work out. However, Youngstedt says, "this could be because people who sleep better in the first place are more willing and able to exercise regularly." It also could be because exercisers typically engage in other habits that are conducive to good sleep, such as avoiding tobacco and limiting caffeine.

If you're an insomniac, don't count out the possibility that working out might offer some relief. Most sleep and exercise studies have focused on good sleepers, so the subjects may simply not have had any room for improvement. Exercise has been shown to have antidepressant and anti-anxiety effects, so it's possible that people who lie awake at night due to anxiety could sleep better if they exercised. And if you're tossing and turning at night, even 10 minutes of extra snooze time is nothing to sneeze at.

## Question #202: Will a hard workout close to bedtime keep me awake?

*The short answer:* It's not likely, although late-night cardio workouts may disrupt sleep for some people.

*If you're all wound up* from a pre-bedtime workout, it seems only logical that you'd be headed for a restless night. But none of the half dozen studies on this topic have found this theory to pan out. In the most extreme example, highly fit men who cycled for three straight hours at 70 percent of their aerobic capacity and finished just 30 minutes before bedtime fell asleep just as quickly and slept just as soundly as they did on a night when they did not exercise. It's possible that trained athletes might be less affected by vigorous late-night workouts than the average person, but research on less fit subjects who worked out for one hour close to bedtime has found similar results.

Still, scientists say, there are probably individual differences in how people respond to pre-bedtime exercise, and some folks might need to exercise earlier in the day. Before you go to the trouble of switching your workout schedule, however, try drinking more fluids during and after your evening workouts. It may be dehydration, rather than the workout itself, that is keeping you up. Also, eating a large meal before bedtime can disturb sleep.

**Question #203: If I don't get enough sleep, will my workouts suffer?**

*The short answer:* Probably not in the short term if you're doing cardiovascular exercise or lifting weights, but researchers haven't studied sports that require coordination and quick thinking, such as tennis or basketball.

*If anxiety about a big swim meet* or bench press competition keeps you tossing and turning all night, don't let concerns about sleep loss compound your worries. Losing one night's sleep doesn't seem to affect strength or aerobic capacity, and some research suggests that staying awake for as long as 60 to 72 consecutive hours doesn't compromise performance. Sleep deprivation may increase your perceived exertion (how tired you feel at various intensity levels); in other words, you might think you're working harder than you really are. However, by most measures, your actual capacity to exercise isn't affected.

Still, the research isn't entirely consistent. While you probably can run or swim just as fast when sleep deprived, some studies suggest that you may tire out about 10 percent sooner than usual. Let's say you're normally able to run at an 8-minute-per-mile pace for 6 miles; you may poop out at about 5.5 miles if you've pulled consecutive all-nighters. Then again, research shows that individuals react in very different ways to sleep deprivation. Some people are able to set personal records on no sleep while others run out of gas.

Most research in this area has looked at one to three nights of complete sleep loss, so it's unclear how night after night of partial sleep deprivation affects athletic performance. But we'd venture a guess that chronic lack of sleep is likely to sap your energy and strength.

**Question #204: How do I know if I've become too obsessed with exercise?**

*The short answer:* Does the thought of missing a workout stress you out? Do you exercise even when you're exhausted or injured? Do you give up social engagements to work out? Do you compulsively monitor your calorie burn? If so, you may have a destructive relationship with exercise.

*Although most Americans* have the opposite problem — they don't exercise *enough* — there are others who are so consumed with working out that they may be damaging their health. Some of the signs of exercise obsession are physical: frequent colds, an elevated resting heart rate, insomnia despite exhaustion, chronic overuse injuries such as stress fractures and tendinitis. But these symptoms — common among athletes who simply train too hard — are also accompanied by low self-esteem, a fear of being fat, and extreme guilt over missing a workout. A person who's obsessed with exercise may feel like a complete failure just because she burned 500 calories when she planned to burn 600.

Exercise obsession often occurs in tandem with food obsession. Sometimes it's symptomatic of an eating disorder, but even people who don't meet the clinical definitions of anorexia or bulimia can still be exercise-obsessed. And like dysfunctional eaters, dysfunctional exercisers ignore signals from their bodies, tuning out pain, fatigue, and hunger. Their main concern is to burn calories. If they miss a workout, all they can think about is how they're going to make up for it, either by doing extra exercise the next day, skipping meals, or both. Because they typically combine excessive exercise with nutritional deprivation, they're often exhausted and irritable and may have trouble concentrating at work or at school.

## Question #205: How can I overcome my obsession with exercise?

*The short answer:* Seeing a therapist, working with a trainer or sports nutritionist, tracking your workouts and fatigue level, reducing your exercise time by small increments — all of these can help you recover from an unhealthy fixation with exercise.

*Like an eating disorder,* an exercise obsession can take a long time to overcome, so you need to be patient with yourself as you try various strategies. Simply recognizing your problem is an enormous step. Many dysfunctional exercisers search high and low for the perfect running-shoe insert or herbal stimulant — anything that will give them back their energy and heal an injury — without even considering that the real problem is that they're exercising too much. Often, it takes a sidelining injury to jolt them into reality.

Counseling from a therapist can help you deal with the personal issues behind your obsession with exercise. A sports nutritionist and/or certified trainer who is knowledgeable about dysfunctional eating and exercise patterns can help educate you about healthy eating and appropriate workout levels.

There are strategies you can try on your own, too. Keep a daily diary to keep a record of how you're feeling — physically and emotionally — before, during, and after your workouts. Also note your eating habits, how long and how well you slept, and how your workday went. Use your diary to make gradual changes. For instance, if you find that you're dragging on Tuesdays after your 8-mile run, cut back, even if it's only by five minutes. People who are truly obsessed with exercise find this assignment tough, but at least making an attempt lets them see how ingrained these habits are.

Try to let go of your magic numbers — for your weight, your swimming yardage, your running distance. Go for a jog without your stopwatch. Go for a bike ride without your cycle computer. Schedule rest into your exercise program. Realize that most serious athletes take one day off a week to rest and refuel their muscles. You might also want to try rewarding yourself with a massage or a shopping trip to diminish the sacrifice you feel you're making when you take a day off.

# Question #206: If I have a history of quitting exercise programs, how can I finally stick with a routine?

*The short answer:* Try a new strategy, like setting a concrete goal, working out with a buddy, joining a club, rewarding yourself, or keeping a workout journal — or try them all.

*Different people get fired up* to exercise for different reasons. For some it's training for a triathlon. For others, it's the thought of squeezing into a swimsuit. But getting motivated is a whole different story than *staying* motivated.

One of the best ways to keep yourself in the groove is to set a specific goal that you can achieve in three to six months while setting steppingstone goals for each month, or even each week, along the way. For instance, if you're aiming to run a 10-k race that's four months away, you may first want to aim for completion of a 5-k distance without stopping or feeling too winded. You can also choose less official goals, like doing 10 full pushups. Your weekly goal could be to do a total-body strength workout twice a week, with emphasis on chest exercises.

If it's weight loss that is motivating you to join a gym or take up cycling, it's a also good idea to set additional goals that have nothing to do with the scale and may ultimately be more satisfying to achieve, like completing a challenging hike or a bike tour in Italy. It's always a good idea to have backup goals in case you get off track from achieving your primary objectives.

If you're really ambitious, you can choose a goal like running a marathon or bicycling a century (100 miles) and join an organized training program such as the Leukemia and Lymphoma Society's Team in Training or similar programs run by the American Diabetes Association or AIDS Rides. These organizations tend to draw many first-timers, so in addition to being coached, you have plenty of people to train with who are at the same fitness level. If you're aiming for a marathon, give yourself six months to one year to train.

Whether or not you're training for an event, working out with a buddy or a club will help keep you accountable and inspired. If you commit to meeting someone at 6 P.M. on Thursday, you're less likely to blow off your workout than if you're accountable to nobody but yourself. Just be sure to choose a buddy who isn't going to blow you off every time she has a hangnail or wants to watch reruns of *Seinfeld*.

A little positive reinforcement also goes a long way. Treating yourself with some small rewards like a bubble bath or a new workout outfit will help you associate exercise with something positive. Just be careful here. Rewarding yourself with a bag of chocolate chip cookies will set you back rather than move you forward.

Tracking your progress in a workout diary is also an excellent motivational tool. Each day, jot down how far or long you exercised. (Note rest days, too, to make sure you're not overtraining.) On Sunday, assess whether you achieved your goals for the week. If you're consistently falling short of your weekly target, you know you need to set more realistic goals — or get moving. If you're consistently meeting or even exceeding your goals, you'll feel the sense of accomplishment, along with the energy and strength, that can transform you into a regular exerciser. Eventually, you'll be one of those people who says, "Sorry, can't watch the football game — gotta go work out!"

## Question #207: What's the best type of exercise for preventing osteoporosis?

*The short answer:* Although scientists are still sorting this issue out, your best bet is combining weight training with weight-bearing aerobic exercise such as walking and jogging. High-impact exercise such as vertical jumping may also help, although it's hard on the joints and risky for people who already have fragile bones.

*As you get older,* it's inevitable that you'll lose bone density. The gradual decline usually starts happening around age 35 and for women it greatly accelerates after menopause. How much bone you lose depends in part on genetics but also on your eating, exercise, and health habits (smokers, for instance, are at greater risk). An estimated 10 million Americans — 80 percent of them women — have lost enough bone mass to develop osteoporosis, also known as brittle bone disease. The disease is responsible for more than 1.5 million fractures a year, primarily at the hip, spine, and wrist.

A diet rich in calcium and vitamin D is essential for maintaining strong bones, but research suggests that exercise also plays an important role in preventing osteoporosis. However, no single type of workout is likely to do the job. Walking may offer some benefits to the spine, although only if it is performed several days a week over the course of several years and at a brisk pace. Jogging and stairclimbing (on actual stairs, not on a machine) appear to do a better job of stimulating bone density at the spine and perhaps the hips than does walking. Swimming and bicycling don't improve bone density, research shows. This is because they don't require lugging your body weight around as you work out.

Lifting weights seems to reduce the risk of fractures in ways that walking and jogging do not. An upper-body routine may help strengthen the wrist bones. Lower-body strength exercises may stimulate bone growth in the spine and hip, as long as you lift sufficiently heavy weights. However, because most studies have lasted just one year, it's unclear how much strength training can do to prevent fractures in the long run.

Recently, researchers have begun investigating the potential benefits of a third type of exercise: high-impact activity such as vertical jumping. Some studies have found dramatic increases in hipbone density after just six months of jumping for two minutes a day. However, researchers caution, high-impact exercise is very hard on the knee and hip joints and risky for people who already have osteoporosis. If you already have low bone density (this can be determined from a low-dose x-ray procedure called DEXA), consult your physician before embarking on any kind of exercise program.

## Question #208: Can exercise help treat clinical depression?

*The short answer:* Yes, aerobic exercise and strength training may be as effective as antidepressants and psychotherapy, at least among patients who are interested in exercise. However, it is important to consult your physician before deciding which approach is best for you.

*The research isn't definitive,* but several studies suggest that regular workouts can help patients with major depressive disorder, a condition with symptoms such as insomnia, fatigue, significant weight loss or weight gain, and feelings of worthlessness. Since 30 to 40 percent of depressed patients don't respond to the first treatment they receive, whether it's drugs or therapy, exercise may be a promising alternative. And it sure costs less.

Studies comparing aerobic exercise to weightlifting have tended to find them equally effective. Relaxation and stretching exercise appear to be less helpful.

Since most studies on exercise and depression have involved group exercise, it's not clear whether the benefit comes from physical exertion or social interaction. Research that has addressed this issue specifically — comparing aerobic workouts to, say, group health seminars or group relaxation classes — suggest that exercise is more useful than social contact alone, although social interaction may help some.

The small amount of research comparing exercise to traditional treatments has found supervised exercise just as useful as therapy and medication. Working out three days a week for 30 minutes at 70 to 85 percent of maximum heart rate seems to be enough. In one study, an exercise-only group showed significantly lower relapse rates than groups that had taken medication or combined medication with exercise.

What makes exercise an apparently useful tool in fighting depression? Regular workouts may trigger chemical changes in the brain, correcting imbalances of neurotransmitters such as serotonin. Or, exercise may boost self-esteem and body image. More likely, it's a combination of these and other benefits.

One caveat: In many exercise studies of depressed patients, only 50 percent of the exercisers stuck with the program for the length of the study. So, exercise clearly isn't the right treatment for everyone diagnosed with depression, nor is it the only treatment. Patients most likely to keep working out, studies suggest, are those who believe in the importance of exercise, who have exercised in the past, who are more fit and knowledgeable about exercise, and who have confidence they can keep up their workouts.

## Question #209: What is Type 2 diabetes, and how does being overweight contribute to it?

*The short answer:* Type 2 diabetes is a disease that results from the body's failure to properly use the hormone insulin. Excess abdominal fat is thought to play a role in triggering the disease, although scientists aren't exactly sure how.

*Type 2 diabetes,* the most common form of diabetes, is often referred to as a "lifestyle disease" because it's almost always associated with being overweight — which is, of course, typically a consequence of being inactive and eating too much. In Type 2 diabetics, either the body does not produce enough insulin or the body's cells ignore the insulin. Insulin is a hormone produced by the pancreas to convert food into energy. More specifically, insulin helps transport glucose — the body's basic fuel — from the blood into the cells. But when this process fails, causing glucose to build up in the blood instead of entering cells, serious problems can result. Left untreated, high blood-sugar levels can damage the eyes, kidneys, nerves, and heart.

Why excess weight sets in motion a cascade of health problems, including diabetes, is not entirely known. But evidence points to visceral fat, the deep fat that resides close to organs. Visceral fat is more "metabolically active" than fat closer to the skin, meaning that it pumps out more byproducts. Among these byproducts are free fatty acids that are dumped directly from the visceral fat into blood vessels leading to the liver. This seems to have a damaging effect not only on the liver but also on many other organs, including the pancreas.

The most successful treatment for Type 2 diabetes seems to be a lifestyle makeover. Losing weight, becoming more active, and eating a calorie-controlled diet that's low in saturated and trans fats and high in fiber seem to be better treatment and prevention strategies than medication, although doctors often prescribe medication when patients can't or won't make changes to their health habits.

About 17 million Americans have diabetes, although about a third of them don't even know it. Some groups are more likely to develop the disease than others. African Americans, Hispanic/Latino Americans, Native Americans, and Pacific Islanders are at particularly high risk for Type 2 diabetes. Not coincidentally, these are also the groups with the highest obesity rates. Experts are also alarmed about double-digit increases in the number of children diagnosed with Type 2 diabetes, which used to be known as "adult-onset diabetes."

Symptoms include frequent urination, excessive thirst, extreme hunger, unusual weight loss, increased fatigue, irritability, and blurry vision. If you suspect you may be diabetic, see a doctor right away. Many of these symptoms don't appear until your blood sugar is really out of whack. If you do experience symptoms on a regular basis. your doctor will run a check called a "fasting glucose" or "fasting blood-sugar" blood test to help determine whether you have diabetes. For more information on diabetes, visit the American Diabetes Association Web site at diabetes.org.

## Question #210: How does Type 1 diabetes differ from Type 2 diabetes?

*The short answer:* Type 1 diabetes is caused by the inability of the pancreas to produce enough insulin for proper sugar regulation.

*Type 1 diabetes* is also known as "juvenile-onset diabetes" because it's generally developed early in life. It's usually hereditary but can also be brought on by poor lifestyle habits or an autoimmune impairment. Between 10 and 15 percent of all diabetics are Type 1.

Some Type 1 diabetics produce no insulin at all, whereas others produce minimal amounts. Either way, they need to inject themselves with insulin several times a day to keep their condition in check. Type 2 diabetics may or may not need to inject insulin.

## Question #211: I keep hearing about Syndrome X and the health problems related to it. What exactly is this condition?

*The short answer:* It's actually a group of conditions that, when occurring together, sharply increase your risk of developing Type 2 diabetes, heart disease, and stroke.

*Although it sounds* like some strange disease contracted by the crew on an old *X-Files* episode, Syndrome X is actually a term coined by a group of researchers at Stanford University to describe a cluster of symptoms, including high blood pressure, high triglycerides (fats in the blood), low HDL (the "good" cholesterol), and abdominal obesity. Although genetics play a significant role in the development of these symptoms, exercise and eating habits are at least as influential, if not more so.

Since Americans are becoming less active and more partial to super-sized portions, it's no surprise that the country has seen a 61 percent increase in Syndrome X in the last decade. About 24 percent of men and 23 percent of women have Syndrome X, according to findings from the third National Health and Nutrition Examination Survey, taken from 1988 through 1994. Using 2000 census data, this means about 47 million Americans have the syndrome. Mexican Americans and African Americans have a higher prevalence than Caucasians. People most likely to be diagnosed with Syndrome X are over 40, have a body mass index greater than 30, and exercise less than three hours a week. Women with a history of pregnancy-related diabetes are also at increased risk.

People with Syndrome X are also insulin resistant, which is why the condition is sometimes referred to as insulin resistance syndrome or metabolic syndrome. Insulin is the hormone responsible for transporting glucose, the body's preferred fuel source, into the body's cells. When you're insulin resistant, your cells don't respond to insulin as well as they should; in other words, they're not as "sensitive" to it. Your body tries to overcome this resistance by churning out extra insulin from the pancreas. Most people can eventually pump out enough insulin to maintain proper blood-glucose levels, but some people cannot. These are the people most susceptible to developing the serious health problems associated with Syndrome X.

The only way to know for sure if you have Syndrome X is to see a doctor for various blood tests. (The chart below lists the criteria for diagnosis.) If you do have the syndrome, you'll probably be advised to limit saturated fats and refined carbohydrates like candy, cake, and soda and to start being more active. You'll also need to lose weight, but research shows it doesn't take that much to make a difference. Losing as little as 5 to 10 percent of your body weight decreases insulin resistance as well as your risk of developing diabetes or heart trouble. If you don't make adequate lifestyle changes, your physician may prescribe medication, but weight loss has been shown to be a far more effective way of controlling the symptoms related to Syndrome X.

### Do I Have Syndrome X?

You may be diagnosed with Syndrome X if you have three or more of the risk factors listed in the following chart. Your doctor can help you interpret the results of your blood tests.

|  | Men | Women |
| --- | --- | --- |
| Waist circumference | >40.2 in. | >34.5 in. |
| Fasting triglycerides | >1.69 mmol/L | >1.69 mmol/L |
| HDL | <1.03 mmol/L | <1.29 mmol/L |
| Blood pressure | 130/85 or greater | 130/85 or greater |
| Fasting glucose | >6.1 mmol/L | >6.1 mmol/L |

Question #212: If I'm overweight, am I at greater risk for developing cancer?

*The short answer:* Yes, excess weight appears to increase the risk of both developing and dying from most types of cancer. In fact, obesity may be responsible for one of every six cancer deaths in the United States — more than 90,000 deaths each year.

*The link between obesity and cancer* is virtually indisputable. In a landmark study published in the *New England Journal of Medicine,* American Cancer Society researchers followed 900,000 people for 16 years, concluding that among people who have never smoked, excess weight may account for 14 percent of all cancer deaths in men and nearly 20 percent of cancer deaths in women. The percentage was higher for women, researchers say, because more women than men are obese and because breast cancer accounts for a large number of cancer deaths among women.

The Cancer Society study substantiated a mountain of previous research linking excess weight to cancers of the colon and rectum, breast (in postmenopausal women), uterus, kidney, esophagus, and gallbladder. In addition, the researchers identified several forms of cancer that had not previously been widely linked to obesity, including stomach (in men), liver, pancreas, prostate, cervical, and ovarian cancers, as well as non-Hodgkins lymphoma and multiple myeloma. The only cancers this study did not link to excess body weight were brain cancer, melanoma, and bladder cancer.

Unlike most other studies, this one looked at *deaths* from cancer, not incidence of the disease. So it's possible that overweight people might not necessarily be at greater risk for developing certain types of cancer but rather they might be more likely to die from the disease because obesity makes cancer harder to diagnose and treat. Excess weight can make it more difficult to see or feel lumps, and some patients don't fit into CAT scanners or radiation-therapy machines. Obese people may also be more likely to avoid regular doctor's visits, and morbidly obese patients are typically more difficult to operate on. In addition, it can be difficult for doctors to choose the right chemotherapy dose for obese patients because fat tissue sometimes absorbs the chemicals.

Body fat can boost the chances of developing cancer in several ways. For women, fat increases the amount of estrogen in the blood, raising the risk of cancers of the female reproductive system. Body fat also increases the risk of acid reflux, also known as heartburn, which can lead to esophageal cancer, and raises insulin levels, prompting the body to create a hormone that causes cells to multiply.

For most obesity-related cancers, the more overweight you are, the greater your risk of dying from the disease. Also, some cancers are more influenced by body weight than others.

## Question #213: Can exercise reduce my risk for cancer even if I'm not overweight?

*The short answer:* There's convincing, although not conclusive, evidence that physical activity reduces the risk for colon cancer and breast cancer. Being active may also lower your risk for prostate, lung, and endometrial cancers. There's not enough research to speculate about the effect of exercise on the risk for developing other forms of cancer.

*There's no question* that maintaining a normal weight lowers your risk for cancer (see Question #212), but staying physically active — regardless of your weight — seems to independently reduce your cancer risk, at least for certain forms of the disease.

The most definitive evidence involves colon cancer. Physically active men and women may be 40 to 50 percent less likely to develop colon cancer than sedentary people. Among the theories explaining the link: Physical activity speeds up the time it takes for food and waste products to make their way through your system, so your colon has less exposure to cancer-causing substances.

The evidence linking physical activity and reduced breast cancer risk isn't as powerful or as consistent as the colon-cancer research, but the case is still fairly strong, suggesting that active women may be 30 to 40 percent less likely to develop breast cancer, probably because physical activity decreases a woman's exposure to estrogen. In men, reduced exposure to testosterone may explain the probable link between exercise and a lower risk for developing prostate cancer.

Exercise may protect against cancer in several other ways, too, such as boosting your immune system, decreasing the amount of insulin circulating in your blood, reducing levels of other hormones, and reducing the amount of fat deep within your belly. (Although you can reduce body fat both by exercising and cutting calories, some research suggests that exercise is more effective than dieting at reducing deep abdominal fat, the most harmful type of fat.)

So how many years — or decades — of exercise does it take to reduce your risk for cancer? How often do you need to break a sweat, how hard do you need to push yourself, and what type of activity works best? Scientists just don't know, in part because studies have used radically different methods for measuring activity levels. In many cases, they've relied on subjects to recall their exercise habits months, years, even decades earlier. For now the best advice is to exercise at least 30 to 45 minutes per day in your target zone (defined in question #119) at least five days a week.

# Mind-Body Exercise: Stretching, Yoga, and Pilates

If you tried to download the last decade's worth of research on weight loss, cardiovascular exercise, and strength training, your hard drive would probably crash. But the sum total of scientific studies conducted on mind-body exercise — including stretching, yoga, and Pilates — would barely eat up a megabyte. Until recently, researchers just haven't paid much attention to these activities.

That doesn't mean mind-body activities aren't as important or as beneficial as other types of workouts. But what the dearth of research does mean is that few definitive assertions can be made, and it can be tough for the consumer to figure out which claims to believe and who's really an expert. Despite the lack of solid information, there's no shortage of hype about the benefits of mind-body exercise. You may be wondering: Will yoga really help you lose weight? Will Pilates give you long, lean muscles? Will stretching prevent injury or muscle soreness?

The questions in this section educate you about what's known and what isn't on the subjects of stretching, yoga, and Pilates. We also explain some basic terms — including exactly what the term *mind-body exercise* means, anyway — and offer tips on how to get started, either on your own or with an instructor. If you don't know your ass from an asana or whether Pilates is a good substitute for lifting weights, you'll find the answers here.

## Question #214: What does the term *mind-body exercise* mean?

*The short answer:* Mind-body refers to any type of exercise that requires a conscious effort to link how you're feeling to what your body is doing.

**Mindful** *is a term that,* when applied to exercise, means taking a thoughtful approach to physical movement. Any type of exercise that you do in a mindful manner can qualify as mind-body, but there are some techniques and activities that have the mindful aspect built in. Yoga and Pilates, for instance, require that you tune in to your body and perform the exercises in a thoughtful manner rather than just go through the motions, as you might do on the stairclimber or a weight machine. Stretching can and should be a mind-body workout.

## Question #215: I have to admit that I don't enjoy stretching. Is it really that important?

*The short answer:* Yes. Stretching is the key to maintaining flexibility, which is pretty darned important whether you're trying to win a limbo contest or simply bending over to tie your shoe. If you don't preserve a certain amount of flexibility in your joints as you age, even hooking a bra or stepping off a curb may pose daunting challenges.

*Superior flexibility* is what allows a prima ballerina to do a perfect *ronde de jambe* and what gives a hurdler the hip flexion he needs to clear a hurdle. It enables a jockey to fold himself tightly into the saddle and a pro football player to twist around to make the game-winning catch. In short, flexibility is one of the elements essential for excelling in sports and fitness. Without good flexibility, athletes, pro and recreational alike, don't have the fluidity to move, bend, jump, run, or curl with ease.

But less athletically inclined people need a certain amount of bendiness, too. When your muscles are stiff and inflexible, it's a lot harder to reach around and grab your wallet off the back seat of your car or bend over to pick up a stack of magazines. You just can't move comfortably without a passable amount of flexibility.

As you age, your tendons (the tissues connecting muscle to bone) begin to shorten and tighten, gradually restricting your flexibility. That's why older folks don't stand up as straight or walk as gracefully as they used to. Flexibility also is crucial to maintaining a sense of balance and coordination — crucial factors, studies show, in preventing falls and keeping that youthful spring in your step. Stretching, like saving for retirement, is one of those things that's easy to neglect but has a critical payoff down the line.

## Question #216: Will stretching make me feel less sore after a workout?

*The short answer:* Probably not. In some cases, stretching may actually intensify muscle soreness.

*The idea that stretching* eliminates soreness gained acceptance in the 1960s, when scientists thought that post-workout aches and pains were caused by deep muscle spasms. Stretching before and after exercise was thought to relax the muscles, thereby calming spasms, thereby relieving soreness.

We now know that muscle soreness is likely caused by microscopic tears in the muscle fibers, not muscle spasms, yet the idea that stretching prevents soreness persists. Dozens of studies have shown that stretching has virtually no influence on how sore you get or how long you remain sore after a workout, regardless of when you stretch, how long you hold a stretch, or how many stretching exercises you do.

In fact, stretching can actually contribute to muscle soreness, especially when you're stiff and tight to begin with. Your body reacts to stretching just as it does to any other form of exercise: When you push your body past the point it's used to being pushed to during the course of a normal day, there's always a chance you'll feel sore for several days afterward. So reaching over and grabbing your toes for a minute or two can be just as seismic an event for your body as a brisk walk if you haven't done it in a while. If you're feeling sore after a workout, you may need to wait a day or two before you stretch.

Does all of this mean stretching is a waste of your time? As we explain in Question #215, of course not. And neither does this mean there's nothing that helps ease the pain of muscle soreness. Flip to Question #198 to find reliable methods for relief of soreness.

## Question #217: Will stretching reduce my risk of injury?

*The short answer:* Nope.

*There are plenty of good reasons* to stretch, but reducing your risk of muscle or joint injury apparently is not one of them. In fact, one large study that compared Dutch army recruits who stretched regularly during military training with recruits who didn't stretch concluded that stretching may prevent one injury every 23 years. Similar studies using a variety of different stretching techniques and flexibility programs have come to similar conclusions.

Some studies have even found that stretching, or at least a high level of flexibility, may even increase your chances of getting hurt. A University of Hawaii investigation that evaluated thousands of runners found that those who had more flexible quadriceps and hamstrings were more likely to develop a serious running injury than their tighter, stiffer counterparts. And super-flexible athletes like dancers, skaters, and gymnasts have incredibly high injury rates. Sure, this may largely be due to the fact that they spend several hours a day doing backflips off balance beams and such, but experts suspect the high injury rates may also, in part, be attributed to excessive flexibility. When a joint is extremely loose, it is also, by definition, very weak, so it may be more susceptible to wear and tear from repetitive activities and to injuries from a single traumatic event, like taking a fall.

## Question #218: Should I stretch at the beginning or the end of my workouts?

*The short answer:* Don't stretch until you have warmed up with at least 3 minutes of cardio exercise. Stretching after your entire workout may be even better.

*Although many people* still start their workouts by tossing one foot up onto a weight bench and reaching for their toes, they're just asking to pull a hamstring muscle or wrench their lower backs.

Stretching a cold, tight muscle is like trying to bend a wooden dowel in half: it's much more likely to snap or break than bend. But warming up with light cardiovascular activity, such as brisk walking or easy pedaling on a bike, sends blood to your muscles, increasing their temperature and making them more supple and pliable. Once a muscle is sufficiently warmed up, stretching is much more pleasant because you can stretch much farther without feeling discomfort.

Although you can warm up and then stretch for a few minutes before continuing on with your cardio or weight-training program, most people prefer to save their stretching until the end of their workout. This is probably the most effective, convenient, and time-efficient way to fit stretching into your routine.

By the way, there is one exception to the no-stretching-before-warming-up rule: active isolated stretching, a technique we describe in Question #220.

## Question #219: How long should I hold a stretch?

*The short answer:* To improve flexibility, one 30-second stretch per muscle group seems to be optimal. Stretching longer than that doesn't appear to be better.

*The American College of Sports Medicine* recommends holding each stretch between 10 and 30 seconds, but new evidence suggests these guidelines need some fine-tuning. Researchers at the University of Arkansas examined several different stretching routines to see which one improved flexibility most. Their conclusion: Holding a stretch for 30 seconds offered better results than holding a stretch for 15 seconds. But surprisingly, a once-a-day, 30-second stretch seems to improve flexibility just as well as a 60-second stretch done three times a day. After 12 weeks, both programs produced about a 25 percent improvement in flexibility. Other recent studies support these findings.

It's unclear why more is not necessarily better, but one theory is that muscles are designed to respond to about half a minute of stretching and no more. Once you reach the 30-second mark, receptors in the muscle signal it to stop lengthening as a protective mechanism against ripping and tearing. No additional stretching will lengthen the muscle any further, so you can't expect one marathon stretching session to make up for years of neglect. The only way to make marked improvements in your flexibility is to stretch consistently over a period of months. (Some experts think a muscle's protective mechanism kicks in after only about two seconds. See Question #221 for more information on this hypothesis.)

There's no question that more research needs to be done comparing various stretching routines. Even though experts agree that flexibility is an important part of being fit, stretching has not been as extensively studied as strength training or cardiovascular exercise.

## Question #220: I tend to skimp on my stretching because it's painful. Is there an alternative method I can try?

*The short answer:* You might want to try *active isolated stretching,* known as AI. This involves stretching a muscle for 2 seconds, then tightening the muscle that's opposite the muscle you're stretching, then repeating the whole shebang several times. Another alternative stretching method, PNF, is described in Question #221.

*For the less bendy among us,* traditional stretching — holding a stretch position for 10 to 30 seconds — can be a painful experience. One possible reason is that tight muscles may not respond well to a sustained stretch. When a muscle is stretched too far or too long, it tightens up and springs back upon itself to prevent ripping and tearing, an automatic defense mechanism known as "the stretch reflex."

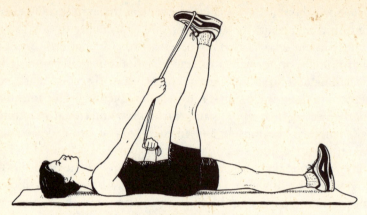

*Active isolated stretches are held for 2 seconds.*

Some experts believe that a good way to avoid discomfort and injuries from overstretching is to steer clear of the stretch reflex by cutting short the duration of the stretch. Active isolated stretching is one method that's based on this theory.

To stretch the AI way, you stretch your target muscle briefly, then tighten the muscle located on the opposite side of the joint, then repeat the process 8 to 12 times. For example, here's how to stretch your quadriceps (front thigh) muscle: In a standing position, bend your left leg behind you and grasp your left toe with your right hand to help pull your heel toward your butt. Hold for 2 seconds to stretch your quadriceps, then let go of your toe and straighten your leg out in front of you to contract the hamstring (rear thigh). Immediately bend your knee and stretch your quads again.

The reason AI may work is that muscles have equal and opposite reactions. When you contract, or shorten, one muscle, the opposite muscle has no recourse but to relax and lengthen. Doing a 2-second stretch may seem counterintuitive, especially since research shows that holding a stretch for 30 seconds is optimal. However, since AI stretches involve continuous movement, they increase blood flow and muscle temperature, ultimately making the muscle more pliable.

AI proponents also claim that this method allows you to isolate one muscle group at a time (traditional stretching tends to stretch several areas of your body at once), so you can zero in and stretch an individual muscle more deeply and thoroughly than you can with traditional stretching. What's more, AI is safe to do as a warm-up before a workout, since all of the movement helps the body prepare itself for more strenuous activity.

So is AI the way to go? There just isn't much scientific information out there that either proves or disproves its effectiveness. No large or long-term studies have done a head-to-head comparison between AI and traditional stretching or between AI and PNF, another alternative stretching method, described in Question #221.

The AI method is gaining popularity among average exercisers and professional athletes alike. We like it, especially for people who are naturally tight and find holding a stretch for 15 to 30 seconds extremely uncomfortable. We know a lot of exercisers who combine AI stretching with conventional stretching. Some do the AI version of an exercise, then hold the last repetition for 30 seconds; others mix the AI stretches that feel the best into their otherwise conventional stretching routine. Both of these are excellent stretching strategies.

The *Whartons' Stretch Book* by Phil and Jim Wharton is a great resource for information about active isolated stretching. Many gyms now offer AI classes or private training sessions. They're sometimes billed as athletic stretch classes.

## Question #221: My trainer recommended PNF stretching. How is this different from regular stretching?

*The short answer:* PNF is a type of stretching that involves three steps: contract, relax, stretch. The theory is that by first tightening the muscle, you exhaust it to the point at which it's too tired to resist being stretched.

*Holy jargon, Batman!* PNF stands for *proprioceptive neuromuscular facilitation*. Thank goodness it's nicknamed PNF. This is the way it works: First you tighten a muscle as much as you can for two or three seconds. Then you relax it, and then you stretch it for

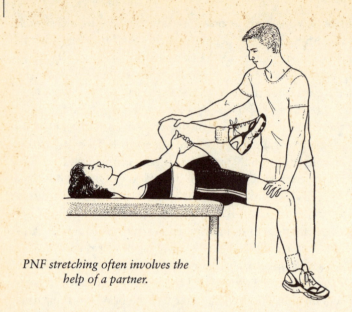

*PNF stretching often involves the
help of a partner.*

about ten seconds. You repeat this five or six times, attempting to stretch a little further each time.

To stretch your hamstring PNF-style, lie on your back with your right leg bent and right foot flat on the floor and your left leg straight and lifted, as close to perpendicular to the floor as you can get it without feeling too much discomfort. Clasp your hands around your left thigh, just below your knee, tighten all of your thigh muscles as hard as you can for a few seconds, and then briefly relax the muscles. Then use your hands to gently pull your thigh closer to your chest.

PNF tends to work best when you have an experienced trainer helping you. For instance, with the hamstring stretch, the trainer can use his weight to gently press your leg toward your chest, pushing a bit farther than you might push yourself.

Is PNF a better way to improve your flexibility than traditional stretching? There's very little research on PNF, but the few studies that have been published suggest that you can get good results this way, and it may even be more effective than conventional stretching. The American College of Sports Medicine seems to think PNF has some value. The organization recommends this type of stretching for people who find conventional stretching painful or ineffective. Despite the shortage of evidence, we agree.

## Question #222: How do the various yoga styles differ?

*The short answer:* Most styles of yoga include roughly the same series of poses, called asanas (pronounced AH-sah-nahs), but they vary in terms of how long you hold each pose, how quickly you move, how much you focus on breathing, and how much of a spiritual element — such as chanting or prayer — is involved. There are more than a hundred types of yoga, so we're just going to mention the most popular. Most of them are offshoots of "hatha" yoga, a branch of yoga that focuses on the physical a bit more than the spiritual.

Most yoga workouts include a blend of strength, flexibility, and body awareness exercises. Classes range from moderately taxing to "Good lord, this instructor has mistaken me for a pipe cleaner," so it's important to choose a school that suits your abilities and fitness level. If you don't like the first class you try, keep looking until you find one that works for you.

### Hatha

The most common type of yoga, hatha, includes all of the basic yoga moves and breathing exercises but doesn't involve the religious or spiritual aspects of some other forms of yoga. Hatha yoga refers to a vast array of beliefs and practices that stress mastery of the physical body as a form of enlightenment. Ananda, Ashtanga, and Bikram are all offshoots of hatha yoga; although most of the poses are the same, the goals, intensity, and pace differ greatly.

### Ananda

Requiring less strength and flexibility than most other yoga styles, Ananda yoga focuses on gentle postures designed to move the body's energy to organs, muscles, and the brain. Classes also emphasize proper body alignment and controlled breathing. Excellent for beginners, Ananda is considered a more meditative approach because each posture is associated with a silent affirmation.

## Ashtanga

Beginners beware: Ashtanga demands significant strength, flexibility, and stamina. This rigorous practice requires moving from one challenging posture to the next without a break, synchronizing each asana with breathing techniques. Each series of poses is done in a precise sequence, and you must master the entire sequence before moving on to the next sequence of poses.

## Bikram

Want to feel like you're working out about seven inches from the sun? Then try Bikram, a strenuous yoga style performed in a room heated up to 105 degrees to mimic the climate of India and promote flexibility. Actually, in our opinion, a better option for most people is simply to choose a different style of yoga. We see no benefit to exercising vigorously in extreme heat, a practice that invites dehydration, if not heat exhaustion. Beginners and anyone with a heart condition should steer very clear of Bikram. Everyone who does try Bikram should drink plenty of water before, during, and after each session. Some instructors may discourage you from bringing a water bottle to class; ignore them. That sort of pressure is not uncommon in Bikram classes, many of which have some decidedly un-yogalike qualities. Whereas most yoga instructors, even the tough ones, create a nurturing atmosphere, Bikram yogis, in our experience, tend to be intimidating and showy, sometimes shouting and bullying class members into various poses.

## Integral Yoga

This approach is basic and straightforward, perfect for beginners and for those who shudder at the thought of going into a full downward dog pose and getting stuck. Integral yoga combines postures, breathing exercises, meditation, chanting, prayer, and self-awareness exercises.

## Iyengar

In an Iyengar class, you hold poses for several minutes and use props such as blankets, straps, and blocks to help you better perform each posture. Ultimately, practitioners strive to perform the postures just as precisely without the props. Iyengar is especially good for anyone looking to improve posture, but since the poses are held for so long, it can be quite an uncomfortable experience if you lack flexibility.

## Kripalu

This gentle, noncompetitive style focuses on taking each pose to your own personal limit. Instructors place a lot of emphasis on regulated breathing and meditation.

## Kundalini

More spiritual than physical, this practice concentrates on awakening the energy at the base of the spine and drawing it upward. In addition to postures, a typical class also includes chanting, meditation, and breathing exercises. If it's too golden-ball-of-light for you, try a more Westernized school of yoga.

## Power Yoga

This is essentially Ashtanga yoga modified for Americans: less chanting, more sweating.

## Urban Yoga

Another form of Americanized yoga, urban classes feature an eclectic mix of flowing postures synchronized to music. They're great for beginners and for anyone who likes a little rock 'n' roll with their sun salutation.

## Question #223: Can yoga help me lose weight?

*The short answer:* Every little bit of exercise helps, but most types of yoga generally don't burn enough calories to be significant tools for weight loss. However, since yoga can have a calming effect, it may help prevent you from raiding the fridge due to stress.

*There's been a proliferation* of "yoga for weight loss" videos and books, and according to yoga philosophy, the postures stimulate your thyroid gland, thereby raising your metabolism and contributing to weight loss. However, there's very little evidence to support the weight-loss claims and none at all to support the notion that yoga revs up your metabolism via stimulated thyroid gland or any other mechanism.

One study done at a meditation school in Sweden investigated the effects of a three-month, comprehensive yoga training program on more than 100 people. Subjects practiced yoga for four hours a day, ate a low-fat vegetarian diet, and worked in the school's garden and fields. Did they lose weight? Yes, of course. Significant amounts. But they didn't just run into their local gym for an express yoga class. You have to wonder how much of the weight loss was due to the yoga and how much was due to their improved dietary habits and exceptionally active lifestyle. You also have to wonder how well they maintained their weight loss after the study was over. Short of moving to the Himalayas, how realistic is this schedule for most of us?

The fact is, while yoga offers many wonderful benefits, a high calorie burn isn't one of them. The average person burns about 240 calories per hour in the typical yoga class. Although this is not an insignificant number — it's about what you'll burn by walking or running 2 miles — you'll probably need to supplement your yoga with cardiovascular activity and improved eating habits to see real weight-loss success.

Sure, you don't see many chubby yoga instructors. But that's because many of them commit to the "yoga lifestyle," which goes way beyond doing a few downward dogs each day. Serious yoga practitioners tend to meditate, walk as much as possible, eat a low-fat, high-fiber vegetarian diet, and engage in other habits that promote a healthy weight. People who commit to this way of life are likely to stay slim whether or not they ever do a cow-face pose.

## Question #224: How do I know if my yoga instructor is qualified?

*The short answer:* Since there are so many styles of yoga and no single certification or even group of certifications is generally recognized as being the best, judging an instructor's credentials can be tough. However, there are clues.

*If a personal trainer* tells you that she is certified by the American College of Sports Medicine, chances are she knows whereof she speaks. But if a yoga instructor tells you she trained for 300 hours with Yogi Master Vishnu Lotusfoot, what are you supposed to make of that? It's a tough call, since there is no gold standard in yoga training, and some of the best instructors may not have a certification that is well-known. With more than 100 types of yoga and countless yoga certification retreats, classes, and weekend workshops, it's a muddy world.

However, standards are emerging. The nonprofit Yoga Alliance, for example, has started a voluntary registration process for teachers who have met certain criteria. The minimum level requires 200 hours of training that includes asana review, anatomy, injury prevention, philosophy, and teaching methodology. More than 3,000 instructors and 137 yoga studios have registered so far. You can use the organization's Web site, yogaalliance.org, to see if your instructor or studio is among them.

An instructor who meets the Yoga Alliance criteria is far more likely to be safe and skilled than someone who has learned yoga from a weekend workshop. But there are plenty of excellent instructors who have not registered, and most certainly inferior yogis who do have the credentials. In the end you're left to judge a yoga instructor based on how well you like her style and personality and what you get out of her class.

If you have more than a casual interest in yoga, you may want to seek out a yoga studio rather than take a yoga class at your health club. Teachers who work for studios typically are very experienced and totally immersed in the yoga lifestyle, so studios are a good place to get deeper into the yoga vibe.

However, this doesn't mean your health club doesn't have perfectly capable yoga instructors. Many instructors split their time between studios and gyms in order to make a living. Some clubs even require their yoga teachers to have a general fitness certification in addition to yoga credentials. This is a nice bonus, but rare is the experienced yoga instructor with mainstream fitness credentials. And a fitness certification won't necessarily make someone a better yoga instructor. Yoga is one of the few cases in which conventional fitness credentials may not translate into a better experience for you. The best yoga teachers tend to be the ones who live, breathe, and study yoga 24-7.

## Question #225: What is Pilates?

*The short answer:* Pilates is an exercise system that was invented around 1900 by Joseph Pilates, a former carpenter and German immigrant to the United States who sought to heal injured dancers and soldiers.

*Joseph Pilates* devised two varieties of exercises. One is a series of yoga-like movements performed on a mat without equipment. The other is a set of moves performed on large contraptions loaded with straps, springs, and handles and carrying exotic names such as the Reformer, the Barrel, and the Cadillac. Mat classes are typically taught to groups, whereas the machines are usually used in one-on-one sessions.

Pilates does a good job of improving flexibility and building moderate amounts of strength. It's especially effective for strengthening your core — your abdominal, lower back, and hip muscles — so it's an excellent exercise regimen for anyone looking to alleviate back pain or improve posture. Although some Pilates and yoga positions are similar, Pilates is much more movement-oriented than yoga. In a properly taught class, you move seamlessly from one exercise to the next. Although a Pilates workout

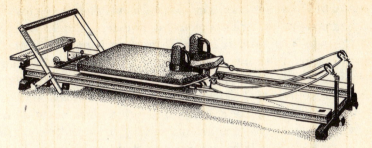

*The Reformer is one piece of specialized equipment used in Pilates.*

can be very challenging — requiring strength, flexibility, and stamina — you usually won't "go to exhaustion," as you would in a weight-training session. Nor would you try to push the limits of your flexibility, as you might in some yoga classes.

Keep in mind that some of the new Pilates systems have changed the basic mat class into something that isn't really Pilates anymore. Instructors may toss in some yoga or ballet or even cardio intervals or weight training. Some of these do a good job of making the complex concepts of Pilates training accessible to the average exerciser. Others are simply parodies of the real thing, with little thought or technique put into the moves.

In addition to taking Pilates classes or getting one-on-one instruction, you can choose from numerous Pilates books and videotapes. You can also purchase scaled-down home versions of professional Pilates machines. As long as you know what you're doing, many of the higher-quality home machines can be quite effective. But we think it's a good idea to take at least a few classes under the watchful eye of an experienced, credentialed Pilates expert before heading off on your own.

## Question #226: Is it true that Pilates will give me long, lean muscles?

*The short answer:* Only if you are predisposed to developing long, lean muscles in the first place.

*You've probably seen ads* with slogans like "Pilates = No Bulk!" or heard claims that Pilates elongates muscles — unlike weight-lifting, which supposedly makes them short and tight. That's a great marketing strategy for Pilates, but it isn't based on any physiological truth. The length of your muscles is dictated by the length of your bones and the way your muscles attach to them. If you have relatively short bones and short, thick muscles, no amount of Pilates will magically stretch your bones or elongate your muscles past their natural potential. In other words, if you're built like a wrestler, don't expect Pilates to turn you into a ballerina. By the same token, if you have relatively long, slender muscles, no amount of weightlifting is going to make them short and thick. (Weightlifting won't make you bulky, anyway, unless you have the genetic predisposition and lift extremely heavy weights.)

Pilates may have gotten this long-and-lean reputation because so many dancers and gymnasts gravitate toward it. In fact, this exercise system was invented specifically to rehabilitate injured dancers. People who excel at doing pirouettes across a stage or rib isolations on the balance beam tend to be lean, willowy types to begin with. The elongated, muscular bodies they develop after a few months of doing Pilates is probably close to how they'd turn out no matter what type of muscle-conditioning program they followed.

That said, Pilates does a good job of stretching your muscles and improving your posture. Anything that helps you stand up straighter and helps you move more fluidly is also bound to give you the appearance of looking taller and leaner. Just don't expect Pilates to transform your body type.

## Question #227: Are yoga and Pilates sufficient for strengthening bones, or do I need to lift weights, too?

*The short answer:* Although hard-core classes may offer almost as much resistance as a moderate weight-training session, most yoga and Pilates workouts don't place enough stress on your bones to help maintain or build bone density, so try to squeeze in two short weight-training sessions a week.

*There are so many styles of exercise* that are good for you that it's darned near impossible to fit them all in. Who has time for weight training, cardio, yoga, Pilates, stretching — and oh yeah, how about tai chi? Since most of us can't devote our entire lives to exercise, it may seem like a smart timesaver — if you enjoy yoga or Pilates — to bypass the weight room. After all, you'll still get a decent muscle-conditioning workout with yoga or Pilates, and in some ways, particularly the emphasis on your core muscles, yoga and Pilates are superior to traditional weight training.

But don't walk away from those dumbbells yet. One thing yoga and Pilates won't do is strengthen your bones. That requires a combination of weight-bearing cardio activity, like walking and jumping, along with strength-training exercises that put a significant amount of stress on your muscles — and therefore your bones. Two 20-minute strength sessions a week will suffice, so you can still lift weights and have plenty of time to perfect your cow-face pose.

## Question #228: Is it okay to do Pilates and weight training on consecutive days? What about yoga and weight training?

*The short answer:* Even though Pilates and yoga don't break down your muscle fibers as much as traditional weight training, and even though these three workouts have different purposes, it's best to give your body a day of rest between a Pilates or yoga workout and a weight-training session.

*If you do a quality Pilates* or yoga workout, your muscles won't be fresh enough to lift weights the next day. Similarly, the day after a weight workout, your muscles will not have recovered enough to put their all into a serious Pilates or yoga routine. (If you feel fully recovered the day after a weight-training session, this means you didn't work as hard as you should have to get all of the muscle-building and bone-strengthening benefits that weight training has to offer.)

However, there are exceptions to this general rule. If the yoga class you take is more on the meditative side or you did a mild Pilates routine that emphasized more stretching than strengthening, it probably won't compromise your weight-training routine the next day. The same holds true if your Pilates or yoga routine focused on certain muscles and your plan is to work an entirely different set of muscles in the weight room. For instance, you might do a series of yoga moves specifically targeted to your abs one day and a lower-body weight-training workout the next.

## Question #229: Can I get an effective Pilates workout on my own, or do I need an instructor?

*The short answer:* Learning Pilates on your own is like learning to knit by reading diagrams; maybe you can muddle your way through it, but you'll progress a lot faster if you spend at least a few hours interacting with an expert.

*To the uninitiated,* Pilates may look like nothing more than a series of movements and positions. Sure, you can see that it requires some flexibility and strength and maybe even a certain level of coordination, but until you've actually done a mat class or a session on the Pilates machines, you can't understand the nuances and precision this technique requires.

It helps to understand the theory behind each move, too. What's the purpose of an exercise like the Seal? Why do you pump your arms up and down as you hold your legs off the floor during the Hundred? How come you flex, then point your foot during the Leg Toss? It takes a knowledgeable Pilates instructor to translate the reasoning, the art, and the science behind the workout. For these reasons, we recommend taking at least a few lessons with a certified teacher before trying Pilates on your own.

## Question #230: Which are the most reputable Pilates certifications?

*The short answer:* Although a recent court decision has led to the proliferation of Pilates certifications, we can recommend just three: the Pilates Guild, TheMethod from the Physicalmind Institute, and Stott Pilates.

*Pilates is a subtle,* nuanced discipline that involves an intricate knowledge of body mechanics and muscle usage. It's not something that you can learn in a weekend workshop, like, say, microwave cooking or flower-arranging basics. A thorough understanding of Pilates and how to teach it comes from hours and hours of study and practical experience. Unfortunately, there are plenty of "certifying" organizations that do not require this level of experience.

Ever since a court decision made Pilates a generic term, an entire industry of 3-day and over-the-Internet Pilates certifications has sprouted up. Now that there is no longer a legal definition of Pilates, it's truly a buyer-beware market. Some large club chains have even slapped together their own certification programs, often staffing their Pilates programs with instructors who've spent more time choosing their workout outfits than studying the art of this discipline. Many instructors change the exercises or teach them incorrectly and simply lack the know-how to give you the true Pilates experience.

Despite all this, there are three major Pilates certifying groups that we know and trust. Here's a rundown of their requirements.

### The Pilates Guild

This group owned the trademark on Pilates until the courts ruled otherwise, and its certification methods are still the gold standard. Requirements include an intensive 12-day seminar that offers hands-on training and instruction in anatomy, physiology, and biomechanics. Within a year of completing this course work, instructors must do at least 600 apprentice hours under the watchful eyes of experienced certified instructors. The tab isn't cheap — training costs at least $3,000 — so instructors have a fairly high level of commitment.

### TheMethod, Physicalmind Institute

This is another of the older, established Pilates schools. Its Concentration certification demands 10 weeks of course work, 275 hours of hands-on experience, and a passing grade on a final written and practical exam. This organization also offers a less stringent Initiation course that requires only a weekend's worth of time, so make sure your instructor has the more demanding certification.

### Stott Pilates

This is a relatively new Pilates school founded by one of the most respected Pilates teachers in the country, Moira Stott. The Comprehensive certification requires extensive course work and 280 hours of practical experience. Like TheMethod, Stott Pilates also offers introductory weekend "certifications."

# Pregnancy: Prenatal Fitness and Postpartum Weight Loss

When you're pregnant, your craving for information about your body and your baby can be even more overwhelming than your craving for salt-and-vinegar potato chips. But advice about exercise can be hard to sort out; urban myths and old wives' tales abound. Can you trust a magazine article that says it's perfectly safe to exercise while you're expecting? Or should you listen to your mother and three aunts who insist that resting up during the nine months was good enough for them and should be good enough for you? Of course, you should always consult your doctor for advice about your own situation, but sometimes the medical community has differing opinions on the subject of pregnancy and exercise, too.

This section addresses the prenatal fitness and postpartum weight-loss questions that women wonder about most: Will working out during pregnancy harm my baby? Can it make my labor and delivery easier? Will I ever be as fit after giving birth as I was before? How long will it take to get my figure back?

Although more studies have been published on some of these topics than others, there's enough research to finally put to rest some of the most persistent myths about pregnancy.

## Question #231: Is it safe to exercise when I'm pregnant?

*The short answer:* Absolutely. Obviously, pregnancy is not the time to take up ice climbing or full-contact karate, but neither do you have to spend nine months parked on the couch knitting booties (unless, of course, you're under doctor's orders). However, since every pregnancy is unique, we recommend working with your doctor to develop workout guidelines best suited for you.

*The first exercise* and pregnancy guidelines issued by the American College of Obstetricians and Gynecologists (ACOG), back in 1985, tended to treat pregnancy as if it were a sickness. There were a lot of absolute "don'ts," and many women found the rules too restrictive. Since then, the body of research on exercise and pregnancy has swelled like a pregnant woman's belly, and it's now clear that exercise does not increase a woman's risk of miscarriage or injury. As a result, ACOG has rethought its recommendations. The most recent guidelines, issued in 1995, are much less limiting.

How hard can you push yourself when preggers? Rate your effort on a scale of 1 to 10, and try to stay in the range of 4 to 8. Experts say that this "perceived exertion" scale (fully explained in Question #125) is more useful during pregnancy than monitoring your heart rate, since your heart rate is affected by so many factors, such as increased blood volume and extra body weight. You'll probably find that you reach the 4-to-8 range a lot more quickly than before you were pregnant, but since you're carrying extra weight that's to be expected.

As for the length of your workout, there are no specific guidelines. This should be based on your pre-pregnancy fitness level, how you feel on a given day and your doctor's recommendations. Just make sure you drink plenty of water before, during, and after you exercise to help keep your system — and the baby's — cool. When you're pregnant, you get dehydrated more easily.

If you were lifting weights before getting pregnant, it's a good idea to continue. If you've never before made the acquaintance of a dumbbell, we recommend you lift weights only under the supervision of an experienced trainer (and, of course, with the permission of your physician). Pay special attention to exercises that work your back and shoulders. Keeping these muscles strong can help counteract the back and shoulder pains that many women experience during pregnancy and ultimately give you more strength to carry around your new bundle of joy, along with the car seat, the stroller, and the jumbo box of Huggies. If you lift

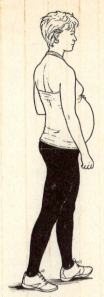

*Staying active during pregnancy will make you feel better.*

weights, do it from a standing, seated, or side-lying position, not while lying flat on your back.

In fact, after the first trimester, you shouldn't do *any* exercises that call for you to lie on your back; you may start feeling dizzy, which means that your little one is pressing on your inferior vena cava, a major vein that carries blood to your heart. So crunches and bench presses are out, but you can — and should — do abdominal exercises from a standing or kneeling position or with your back pressed against a wall.

A stretching routine can also help relieve general aches and pains, but don't push beyond the point of mild discomfort or hold the stretches longer than 20 seconds. When you're pregnant you produce more of a hormone called relaxin, so your joints are a bit looser than normal, and pushing stretches too far can lead to permanent injuries. Be especially careful when you stretch the muscles that surround your knees, hips, and lower back.

Consider taking a prenatal exercise class, whether it's aerobics, stretching, or yoga. The moves are customized for pregnant women's morphing bodies, and it's a great way to lessen that "Am I the only woman who can't dress like a Barbie doll?" feeling.

The general rule for exercise and pregnancy: If it doesn't feel good, skip it. Some women continue running well into late pregnancy. Others find they don't have enough energy or feel too awkward to continue their usual workouts so they back off, although most women find walking and swimming doable right up to the day they give birth. If you can't do your regular routine, don't get discouraged. Better to switch gears and maintain fitness any way you can, since women who are in better shape — no matter how they get there — usually bounce back more quickly after delivery.

## Question #232: If I exercise while I'm pregnant, will I have an easier labor?

*The short answer:* The odds appear to be in your favor if you exercise, although there are certainly no guarantees.

*There hasn't been* a heckuva lot of research in this area and results have been mixed. However, studies do suggest that women who begin pregnancy in good shape and continue aerobic exercise for the whole nine months tend to have easier, shorter, and less complicated labors than women who don't work out.

One study compared pregnant non-exercisers with fit pregnant women who did weight-bearing exercise (such as walking, as opposed to cycling or swimming) at least three times a week for at least 30 minutes. The results were dramatic: Whereas 78 percent of the non-exercisers needed pain-relief medication, only 51 percent of the exercisers did. The fit women were 50 percent less likely to have labor induced, and 55 percent less likely to need an episiotomy (a cut between the vagina and rectum to give the baby more room). Only 9 percent of the exercisers had cesarean sections, compared with 29 percent of the women who didn't work out.

Among the women who gave birth vaginally, the exercisers experienced labors that were one-third shorter than the labors of the non-exercisers. More than 65 percent of the exercising women delivered in less than 4 hours, compared with 31 percent of the non-exercisers. All the fit women gave birth in less than 10 hours, whereas 15 percent of the control group had active labor lasting between 10 and 14 hours. Although other studies have shown no difference in the length or ease of labor between exercising and unfit women, these results are impressive because the researchers tracked the women all the way through their pregnancies and were actually present during labor to document what went on.

Still, even world-class athletes have experienced labors more grueling than an Olympic heptathlon. So although the odds might favor quicker, easier deliveries for fit women, there are no certainties when it comes to childbirth.

# Question #233: Will I gain less weight during pregnancy if I exercise?

*The short answer:* Probably, as long as you exercise at least three days a week throughout your pregnancy.

*In the first half of pregnancy,* pregnant women who do aerobic exercise gain about the same amount of weight as women who don't work out. But research suggests there are dramatic differences in the final 20 weeks. In one study of 75 pregnant women, those who exercised at least three days a week for at least 30 minutes gained on average 7 pounds less than women who either didn't exercise or stopped working out early in pregnancy. The more women exercised, the less weight they gained, although all of the exercising women were well within the normal, healthy range of weight gain, putting on an average of 29 pounds.

All of the exercisers in that study worked out regularly before getting pregnant. Research suggests that people who start an exercise program after getting pregnant need to exercise more — a total of at least three hours a week, perhaps more — to achieve the same benefits as women who were already fit when they conceived.

# Question #234: Will I ever be as fit after pregnancy as I was before?

*The short answer:* Actually, research suggests you may have the capacity to be even more fit after pregnancy, although how well you actually perform depends in large part on your workout program.

*There's no shortage of stories* about elite runners who have gone on to win races and set personal records after giving birth. In 1983, Norway's Ingrid Kristiansen won the Houston marathon five months after giving birth to a son; two years later, she set a world record in the London marathon. In the 1996 Olympics, Svetlana Masterkova of Russia won the 800-meter and 1,500-meter races about a year after delivering a daughter, then broke the world record for the mile a few months later. Sprinter Valerie Brisco, who won three gold medals in the 1984 Olympics, when her son was one year old, told the media that pregnancy "is better for you than a store full of vitamins or steroids or anything else."

Certainly, pregnancy isn't going to work wonders for everyone, and no one is recommending it as a method of shaving 3 minutes off your 10-k time. But if you're an athlete or avid exerciser who's concerned that getting pregnant will doom your athletic career, research suggests that's not the case.

Studies have found a small but significant increase in maximal aerobic capacity, a.k.a VO2 max (defined in Question #128), in well-trained women who maintain a moderate to high level of training during and after pregnancy. In one study of 20 pregnant runners and cross-country skiers, VO2 max remained elevated until the end of the testing period, 11 months postpartum. The authors concluded that the combination of exercise and pregnancy may have a greater training effect than exercise alone, probably due to the increase in blood volume and changing hormone levels. In other words, the adaptations your body must make to carry the extra — and constantly increasing — load may, in some respects, simulate a workout.

Of course, just because you may have the potential to achieve a postpartum personal best doesn't mean it will happen. While the demands of pregnancy may make you fitter, the demands of momhood may lead you in the opposite direction. With the addition of precious little ones to their lives, many women don't have as much time or motivation to train at the same level they used to.

## Question #235: Will working out affect how much breast milk I produce or what it tastes like to my baby?

*The short answer:* Exercise won't compromise your breast-milk production. Although extremely intense exercise sometimes makes breast milk taste sour due to a higher concentration of lactic acid, infants generally accept milk even after mom has done a vigorous aerobic workout.

*Sometimes rumors* can spread on the basis of a single study testing an extreme set of circumstances. That's essentially what happened some years back, when a study found that infants were significantly less accepting of their mothers' breast milk 30 minutes after the moms had run on the treadmill. Apparently, the taste of the milk had been altered by elevated levels of lactic acid (defined in Question #126), which is produced at high levels by the body during strenuous exercise. But here's what got lost in some reports on the study: The women had pushed as hard as they possibly could, crossing the line from aerobic to anaerobic exercise (defined in Question #113).

Plenty of other studies have concluded that moderate to vigorous exercise that falls short of an all-out effort doesn't elevate lactic acid levels enough to alter the taste of breast milk. With occasional exceptions, even lactating athletes who train at high levels for more than an hour almost daily seem to have no problems breastfeeding.

## Question #236: Will I lose weight more quickly if I breastfeed my baby than if I bottlefeed?

*The short answer:* Probably, but the difference isn't huge — about 1½ to 4½ pounds over the course of a year. When it comes to postpartum weight loss, your eating habits and physical activity level play a more important role in weight loss than whether or not you nurse your baby.

*In theory, breastfeeding* should be a major boon for weight loss. For the first six months after giving birth, women who feed their infants only breast milk burn on average 595 to 670 extra calories a day. That adds up to a whopping 117,000 more calories than a bottlefeeding mom — enough, theoretically, for a nursing mother to lose about 28 pounds of fat. Yet some studies show that breast-feeding women have no weight-loss advantage over those who bottlefeed, and other studies show only a small benefit. What gives?

Basically, breastfeeding moms tend to compensate for the extra calorie burn by eating more than women who bottlefeed. Still, there does appear to be some weight-loss advantage to nursing, even if it's not as great a bonus as you might expect. According to the most carefully conducted studies, women who feed their babies nothing but breast milk lose a few more pounds than their bottlefeeding counterparts, primarily between three and six months postpartum. Before and after that period, however, there appears to be less of a weight-loss benefit.

The prevailing theory is that in the first few months postpartum, nursing moms have very high concentrations of prolactin, a hormone that stimulates breast-milk production and also stimulates appetite. After about three months, prolactin levels typically decline, even if a woman is still producing plenty of milk, so it only makes sense that a woman's appetite would decline, too. After six months, particularly when complementary solids are added to the baby's diet, nursing mothers tend to produce less breast milk than before, so they're burning fewer calories — hence the reduced advantage of breastfeeding.

In addition to promoting weight loss, breastfeeding has countless other benefits, including nutritional and immune-boosting advantages for your baby. Just keep in mind that nursing is not an express ticket to regaining your pre-pregnancy body. Some women actually gain weight while breastfeeding, perhaps because they're hungrier and less active than some women who bottlefeed.

## Question #237: What's the best way to lose weight after pregnancy?

*The short answer:* Watch what you eat, exercise, and be patient — the same advice that applies to everyone, whether they've had a baby or not.

*Exercise is important* for postpartum weight loss — it will help you preserve lean tissue as you lose fat — but research shows you can't count on workouts alone to help you slim down after giving birth. In one study of new moms, those who exercised five days a week for 45 minutes — burning, on average, 400 calories per workout — did not lose any more weight after 12 weeks than women who didn't exercise. Why not?

Because the exercising women, like subjects in other studies, compensated for the calories burned during their workouts, either by eating more or becoming less active when they weren't exercising. One possible way to avoid falling into this trap: Be active with your baby. Dance with her in your arms when she's younger, then run around with her once she's mobile.

Be patient: Whether you're breastfeeding or not, it generally takes six months to a year to return to your pre-pregnancy size. However, losing all of the weight you've gained isn't a given. As we explain in Question #238, many women end up heavier after pregnancy than they were before. Whether — and how quickly — you slim back down depends on your eating and exercise habits as well as the amount of weight you gained during pregnancy. Typically, the more weight you have to lose, the longer it'll take.

## Question #238: Will I gain weight permanently after having a baby?

*The short answer:* That depends in large part on whether you exercise during and after pregnancy.

*First, the good news.* Women who are fit when they become pregnant, do aerobic exercise more than three days a week for at least 20 minutes all the way through pregnancy, and keep up their routines afterward tend to weigh the same five years after giving birth as they did before getting pregnant. But that scenario doesn't describe most women.

In general, women do tend to be heavier after giving birth — and how much heavier seems to correlate directly with how much weight they gain while pregnant. In one study of 500 women, researchers found that eight and a half years after giving birth, mothers who gained more than the recommended amount of pregnancy weight had put on 18.5 pounds, compared with 14.3 pounds for those who gained the recommended amount of weight (typically 25 to 35 pounds for women at a healthy weight and 15 to 25 pounds for overweight women). The women who gained less weight than the guidelines recommended were, on average, 9 pounds heavier than before getting pregnant.

However, a small percentage of the women in the study gained no weight at all, and researchers found that the women who gained the least amount of weight were the ones who breastfed their children for at least six months and who did aerobic exercise consistently.

Researchers say that the pounds probably pile up for a variety of reasons. It could be that moms tend to have less time for themselves, so they exercise less, or that they eat more and make more impulsive, less healthy food choices. They may have more than one child, which can equate to even more pregnancy-associated weight gain and even less "me" time.

On the other hand, research shows, moms who continue to work out through two pregnancies are, on average, lighter and leaner before their second pregnancy than they were before their first.

## Question #239: How soon after I give birth can I start exercising again?

*The short answer:* Some women practically jump up and head to the nearest aerobics class a few days after giving birth, whereas others don't feel up to moving and sweating for several weeks. Some women, particularly those who have had cesarean sections, will need to wait longer than others before getting back in the exercise groove.

*You're exhausted,* exhilarated, overwhelmed, overjoyed — those first few weeks of momhood are like no others, and working out may be the farthest thing from your mind. Still, it's important to begin exercising as soon as you're safely able to. It can be a wonderful way to carve out some much-needed time for yourself and begin reclaiming your body.

Few scientific investigations have delved into the optimal time to begin exercising after you've had a baby, but even if there were scads of research, it wouldn't change the fact that every woman has a unique prenatal and postpartum experience. You can't hit the gym or break out the exercise videos until you feel up to it and, of course, until you get the green light from your doctor.

As a general rule, most women are able to do some light activity within six weeks after giving birth. If you've had a cesarean delivery, plan on taking a little longer. Your abdominal wall has been sliced through and requires time to heal, so naturally you'll need to take more precautions and ease into an exercise program more slowly than someone who has had an uncomplicated vaginal delivery.

Brisk walking is a good place for most new moms to start. If you've had an episiotomy, your doctor will probably tell you cycling is out. Report any abnormal, exercise-associated pain or heavy bleeding (bright-red bleeding that persists for several hours) to your doctor.

If you were an avid exerciser before you got pregnant, don't expect to dive right back in at the same level. Start slowly. Whatever your program, make sure to drink plenty of fluids, wear a supportive bra (or even two), and, if possible, wear some Lycra tights to hold in your abdominals, which are probably somewhat lax from giving birth.

And remember: You didn't create your baby in a day, so don't expect your body to snap back to its old self in a day, either. It may take a while before the baby fat begins to peel off and you're back exercising at your old level again. Don't be too hard on yourself if you don't look exactly the way you did before your baby was born. After all, look what you have to show for it.

# Where to Go
# from Here

If there's one constant about fitness and nutrition, it's that there's nothing constant. There's always going to be some new diet or exercise gizmo or weight-loss trend in the making. So how can you evaluate the new products, programs, and theories you come across? What steps can you take to distinguish the schlock from the sure thing?

You can start by relying on common sense and trusting your instincts. Of course, not all rip-offs or bad ideas are obvious, but it doesn't take a degree in kinesiology to figure out that you can't transform your body by exercising 10 minutes a week, even if the "doctor" on the infomercial says otherwise.

Try to put new information into context, especially the stuff that gets hyped in the media. Ask yourself: How does the latest low-carb diet study compare to the studies that came before it? The results of a single research trial may provide only a tiny piece of a complex puzzle, so don't change your lifestyle based on its outcome.

It's especially important to consider the source of the information you hear. Was the "stunning new research" published in a legitimate scientific journal, or was it the product of a clever marketing campaign? The organizations listed on page 319 can help you continue your quest for honest information. You can check in with them periodically to see what's new. Or, you can use them to research a specific topic, whether it's treadmills, trans fats, or target heart-rate zones. The more sources you explore and the more questions you ask, the more likely you are to locate the truth.

Aerobics and Fitness Association of America
afaa.com

American College of Obstetricians and Gynecologists
acog.org

American College of Sports Medicine
acsm.org

American Council on Exercise
acefitness.org

American Diabetes Association
diabetes.org

American Dietetic Association
eatright.org

American Society of Bariatric Physicians
asbp.org

Center for Science in the Public Interest
cspinet.org

Federal Trade Commission
ftc.gov

Food and Drug Administration
fda.gov

Institute of Medicine of the National Academies
iom.edu

National Academy of Sports Medicine
nasm.org

National Institutes of Health
nih.gov

National Strength and Conditioning Association
nsca-lift.org

National Weight Control Registry
uchsc.edu/nutrition/Wyatt Jortberg/nwcr.htm

U.S. Department of Agriculture's National Nutrient Database for Standard Reference
nal.usda.gov/fnic/foodcomp/search/

Yoga Alliance
yogaalliance.org

# Sources

## Question #3: Are Americans really that much fatter than they used to be?

National Center for Health Statistics. Results from the 1999–2000 National Health and Nutrition Examination Survey (NHANES), cdc.gov/nchs/products/pubs/pubd/hestats/obese/obse99.htm.

## Question #4: How much less active are we compared to our pre-modern ancestors?

1. Garry J. Egger, Neeltje Vogels, and Klaas R. Westerterp, "Estimating historical changes in physical activity levels," *Medical Journal of Australia*, v. 175, 2001, pp. 635–636.
2. David Bassett et al., "Physical activity in an Old Order Amish community," *Medicine & Science in Sports & Exercise*, v. 36, January 2004, pp. 79–85.

## Question #5: Are Americans the fattest people in the world?

International Obesity Task Force, The Global Epidemic of Obesity, data from various published sources, iotf.org.

## Question #6: To what extent is my weight influenced by my genes?

1. Claude Bouchard, Angelo Tremblay, et al., "The response to long-term overfeeding in identical twins," *New England Journal of Medicine,* v. 322, May 24, 1990, pp. 1478–1482.
2. Claude Bouchard, Angelo Tremblay, et al., "Overfeeding in identical twins: 5-year postoverfeeding results," *Metabolism,* v. 45, 1996, pp. 1042–1050.
3. Albert J. Stunkard, Jennifer R. Harris, et al., "The body-mass index of twins who have been reared apart," *New England Journal of Medicine,* v. 322, May 24, 1990, pp. 1483–1487.

**Question #7: Am I destined to gain fat and lose muscle mass as I get older?**

Kent Adams, Patrick O'Shea, Katie O'Shea, "Aging: Its effects on strength, power, and bone density," *Strength and Conditioning Journal,* v. 21, April 1999, pp. 65–76.

**Question #11: If I gain weight, will I gain fat cells or will the ones I have expand?**

W. C. Chumlea, A. F. Roche, et al., "Adipocytes and adiposity in adults," *American Journal of Clinical Nutrition,* v. 9, September 1981, pp. 1798–1803.

**Question #16: I seem to weigh more when my scale is on a carpet than when it's on tile. Am I imagining this?**

Ian Sample, "Rip up the shag pile if you want to lose weight," *New Scientist,* v. 174, June 2002, p. 23.

**Question #22: What is the strongest muscle in the body?**

*Guinness Book of World Records* (New York: Bantam Books, 1995), p. 24.

**Question #33: Which cardio machine burns the most calories?**

Barbara Ainsworth et al., "The Compendium of Physical Activities Tracking Guide: An update of activity codes and MET intensities," *Medicine & Science in Sports & Exercise,* v. 32 (Supplement), 2000, pp. S498-S516.

**Question #34: Will I burn as many calories running on the treadmill as I do running outdoors?**

Barbara Ainsworth et al., "The Compendium of Physical Activities Tracking Guide: An update of activity codes and MET intensities," *Medicine & Science in Sports & Exercise,* v. 32 (Supplement), 2000, pp. S498–S516.

**Question #35: Can I trust the calorie counters on exercise equipment?**

A. C. Utter, D. C. Nieman, et al., "Influence of diet and/or exercise on body composition and cardiorespiratory fitness in obese women," *International Journal of Sport Nutrition and Exercise Metabolism,* v. 8, September 1998, pp. 213–222.

**Question #36: Will I burn more calories if I carry hand weights while walking?**

Len Kravitz et al., "Does step exercise with handweights enhance training effects?" *Journal of Strength and Conditioning Research,* v. 11, 1997, pp. 194–199.

**Question #37: Will I burn more calories running on the beach than on the street?**

Barbara Ainsworth et al., "The Compendium of Physical Activities Tracking Guide: An update of activity codes and MET intensities," *Medicine & Science in Sports & Exercise,* v. 32 (Supplement), 2000, pp. S498–S516.

**Question #38: I hear jumping rope is one of the best ways to burn calories. Just how effective is it?**

Barbara Ainsworth et al., "The Compendium of Physical Activities Tracking Guide: An update of activity codes and MET intensities," *Medicine & Science in Sports & Exercise,* v. 32 (Supplement), 2000, pp. S498–S516.

**Question #39: Will I burn more calories exercising in hot or cold weather?**

Barbara Ainsworth et al., "The Compendium of Physical Activities Tracking Guide: An update of activity codes and MET intensities," *Medicine & Science in Sports & Exercise,* v. 32 (Supplement), 2000, pp. S498–S516.

**Question #40: Will I burn more calories on a stairclimbing machine or climbing real steps?**

Barbara Ainsworth et al., "The Compendium of Physical Activities Tracking Guide: An update of activity codes and MET intensities," *Medicine & Science in Sports & Exercise,* v. 32 (Supplement), 2000, pp. S498–S516.

**Question #42: Will regular cardio exercise boost my resting metabolism?**

Richard C. Bullough, Cynthia A. Gillette, et al., "Interaction of acute changes in exercise energy expenditure and energy intake on resting metabolic rate," *American Journal of Clinical Nutrition,* v. 61, March 1995, pp. 473–481.

**Question #43: Can weight training rev up my metabolism?**

Eric T. Poehlman, Christopher Melby, "Resistance Training and Energy Balance," *International Journal of Sport Nutrition and Exercise Metabolism,* v. 8, June 1998, pp. 143–159.

**Question #44: Is it true that my metabolism stays elevated after a workout?**

Cynthia A. Gillette, Richard C. Bullough, et al., "Postexercise energy expenditure in response to acute aerobic or resistive exercise," *International Journal of Sport Nutrition and Exercise Metabolism,* v. 4, December 1994, pp. 347–360.

**Question #45: If I had anorexia, is my metabolism permanently damaged?**

J. Russell, L. A. Baur, et al., "Altered energy metabolism in anorexia nervosa," *Psychoneuroendocrinology,* v. 26, January 2001, pp. 51–63.

**Question #48: Which is more important for weight loss, diet or exercise?**

1. John M. Jakicic, "American College of Sports Medicine position stand. Appropriate intervention strategies for weight loss and prevention of weight regain for adults," *Medicine & Science in Sports & Exercise,* v. 33, December 2001, pp. 2145–2156.
2. R. D. Hagan, S. J. Upton, et al., "The effects of aerobic conditioning and/or caloric restriction in overweight men and women," *Medicine & Science in Sports & Exercise,* v. 18, 1986, pp. 87–94.
3. "Clinical Guidelines on the identification, evaluation, and treatment of overweight and obesity in adults: the evidence report," NIH Publication No. 98-4083, National Institutes of Health, 1998.

**Question #50: What's the best way to reduce a paunchy middle?**

M. L. Irwin, Y. Yasui, et al., "Effect of exercise on total and intra-abdominal body fat in postmenopausal women," *Journal of the American Medical Association,* v. 289, January 2003, pp. 323–330.

### Question #52: Will yo-yo dieting make me fatter?

1. National Task Force on the Prevention and Treatment of Obesity, "Weight cycling." *Journal of the American Medical Association,* v. 272, October 1994, pp. 1196–1202.
2. A. E. Field, S. B. Austin, et al., "Relation between dieting and weight change among preadolescents and adolescents," *Pediatrics,* v. 112, October 2003, pp. 900–906.

### Question #55: I've heard that swimming isn't as effective for weight loss as other forms of exercise. Is this true?

1. Georgianna Tuuri, Mark Loftin, Jeffrey Oescher, "Association of swim distance and age with body composition in adult female swimmers," *Medicine & Science in Sports & Exercise,* v. 34, December 2002, pp. 210–214.
2. M. G. Flynn, D. L. Costill, et al., "Fat storage in athletes: Metabolic and hormonal responses to swimming and running," *International Journal of Sports Medicine,* v. 11, December 1990, pp. 433–440.
3. Grant Gwinup, "Weight loss without dietary restriction: Efficacy of different forms of aerobic exercise," *American Journal of Sports Medicine,* v. 15, May–June 1987, pp. 275–279.

### Question #56: Does menopause cause women to gain weight?

1. M. L. Irwin, Y. Yasui, et al., "Effect of exercise on total and intra-abdominal body fat in postmenopausal women," *Journal of the American Medical Association,* v. 289, January 2003, pp. 323–330.
2. Eric T. Poehlman, Michael J. Toth, et al., "Changes in energy balance and body composition at the menopause: a controlled longitudinal study," *Annals of Internal Medicine,* v. 123, November 1995, pp. 673–675.
3. Michael J. Toth, André Tchernof, et al., "Menopause-related changes in body fat distribution," *Annals of the New York Academy of Science,* v. 904, May 2000, pp. 502–506.

### Question #58: I've noticed that a lot of people gain weight after they get married. Is there any correlation?

1. Jeffery Sobal, Barbara Rauschenbach, Edward A. Frongillo, "Marital status changes and body weight changes: A U.S. longitudinal analysis," *Social Science & Medicine,* v. 56, April 2003, pp. 1543–1555.

2. Robert W. Jeffery, Allison M. Rick, "Cross-sectional and longitudinal associations between body mass index and marriage-related factors," *Obesity Research,* v. 10, August 2002, pp. 809–815.

**Question #60: If a dietary supplement claims to "assist with weight loss" or "reduce fat absorption," how do I know if it's true?**

1. U.S. Food and Drug Administration, Center for Food Safety and Applied Nutrition, Dietary Supplements: Overview, cfsan.fda.gov/~dms/supplmnt.html.
2. Marion Nestle, *How the Food Industry Influences Nutrition and Health* (Berkeley: University of California Press, 2002), pp. 223–236.
3. "Report on Weight-Loss Advertising: An Analysis of Current Trends," Federal Trade Commission, September 2002, ftc.gov/opa/2002/09/weightlossrpt.htm.

**Question #63: Even though ephedra has been banned by the federal government, many people are still taking it. Is ephedra really unsafe?**

Paul G. Shekelle, Mary L. Hardy, "Efficacy and safety of ephedra and ephedrine for weight loss and athletic performance," *Journal of the American Medical Association,* v. 289, March 26, 2003, pp. 1537–1545.

**Question #64: Can ephedra help me lose weight or improve my athletic performance?**

Paul G. Shekelle, Mary L. Hardy, "Efficacy and safety of ephedra and ephedrine for weight loss and athletic performance," *Journal of the American Medical Association,* v. 289, March 26, 2003, pp. 1537–1545.

**Question #66: How do prescription weight-loss drugs work?**

J. Cerulli, "Update on the pharmacotherapy of obesity," *Annals of Pharmacotherapy,* v. 32, January 1998, pp. 88–102.

**Question #67: How effective are prescription weight-loss drugs?**

1. G. A. Bray, D. H. Ryan, et al., "A double-blind randomized placebo-controlled trial of sibutramine," *Obesity Research,* v. 4, 1996, pp. 263–270.
2. N. V. Dhurandhar, "Initial weight loss as a predictor of response to obesity drugs," *International Journal of Obesity and Related Metabolic Disorders,* v. 23, December 1999, pp. 1333–1336.

3. S. Rossner, L. Sjostrom, R. Noack, et al., "Weight loss, weight maintenance, and improved cardiovascular risk factors after 2 years' treatment with orlistat for obesity," *Obesity Research,* v. 8, 2000, pp. 49–61.
4. T. A. Wadden, R. I. Berkowitz, et al., "Benefits of lifestyle modification in the pharmacologic treatment of obesity," *Archives of Internal Medicine,* v. 161, 2001, pp. 218–227.

### Question #68: How safe are weight-loss drugs?

T. A. Wadden, R. I. Berkowitz, et al., "Benefits of lifestyle modification in the pharmacologic treatment of obesity," *Archives of Internal Medicine,* v. 161, 2001, pp. 218–227.

### Question #71: What's the success rate of weight-loss surgery?

Louis Flancbaum, Erica Manfred, Deborah Biskin, *The Doctor's Guide to Weight Loss Surgery: How to Make the Decision That Could Save Your Life* (New York: Fredonia Communications, 2001).

### Question #72: How do I know if I'm a good candidate for weight-loss surgery?

Louis Flancbaum, Erica Manfred, Deborah Biskin, *The Doctor's Guide to Weight Loss Surgery: How to Make the Decision That Could Save Your Life* (New York: Fredonia Communications, 2001).

### Question #80: I heard that obesity can be caused by a virus. Could this possibly be true?

1. N. V. Dhurandhar, "Infectobesity: obesity of infectious origin," *Journal of Nutrition,* v. 131, October 2001, pp. 2794S–2797S.
2. N. V. Dhurandhar et al., "Transmissibility of adenovirus-induced adiposity in a chicken model," *International Journal of Obesity and Related Metabolic Disorders,* v. 25, July 2001, pp. 990–996.

### Question #81: What is leptin, and what does it have to do with weight loss?

1. Paul Cohen, Connie Zhao, et al., "Selective deletion of leptin receptor in neurons leads to obesity," *Journal of Clinical Investigation,* v. 108, October 2001, pp. 1113–1121.

2. A. Chen et al., "Inactivation of the mouse melanocortin-3 receptor results in increased fat mass and reduced lean body mass, *Nature Genetics,* v. 26, September 2000, pp. 97–102.

3. C. T. Montague et al., "Congenital leptin deficiency is associated with severe early-onset obesity in humans," *Nature,* v. 387, June 26, 1997, pp. 903–908.

### Question #82: How do sumo wrestlers get so fat, and how unhealthy are they?

A. Hoshi, Y. Inaba, "Risk factors for mortality and mortality rate of sumo wrestlers," *Nippon Eiseigaku Zasshi,* v. 50, August 1995, pp. 730–736.

### Question #85: For weight loss, is it better to eat six small meals a day than three large ones?

F. Bellisle, R. McDevitt, et al., "Meal frequency and energy balance," *British Journal of Nutrition,* v. 77 (Supplement 1), April 1997, pp. S57–S70.

### Question #90: Can I trust the labels on supermarket foods or the calorie counts listed on chain-restaurant Web sites?

1. Mitch Lipka, "Many food labels are incorrect: Errors in 'Nutritional Facts' panels may be hazardous to health of consumers," *South Florida Sun-Sentinel,* September 2, 2001, p. 1A.

2. Mitch Lipka, "Brazen deceit produces jail term: Low-calorie claims drew FDA inquiry," *South Florida Sun-Sentinel,* September 9, 2001, p. 6A.

3. Tests commissioned by the Center for Science in the Public Interest: "'Laura's Lean' steaks fattier than labeled," April 1, 2003, cspinet.org/new/200304011.html.

### Question #91: Are portion sizes larger than they used to be?

1. Lisa R. Young, Marion Nestle, "Expanding portion sizes in the U.S. marketplace: Implications for nutrition counseling," *American Journal of Public Health,* v. 92, February 2002, pp. 246–249.

2. American Institute for Cancer Research, "New survey shows Americans ignore importance of portion size in managing weight," March 31, 2000, aicr.org/presscorner/pubsearchdetail .lasso?index=152.

**Question #92: If I'm trying to lose weight, what's the maximum amount of fat I should eat each day?**

1. Walter C. Willet, Rudolph L. Leibel, "Dietary fat is not a major determinant of body fat," *American Journal of Medicine,* v. 113, December 2002, pp. 47S–59S.
2. John P. Foreyt, Walker S. Carlos Poston II, "Consensus view on the role of dietary fat and obesity," *American Journal of Medicine,* v. 113, December 2002, pp. 60S–62S.
3. Susan B. Roberts, Megan A. McCrory, Edward Saltzman, "The influence of dietary composition on energy intake and body weight," *Journal of the American College of Nutrition,* v. 21, April 2002, pp. 140S–145S.

**Question #93: Is a low-fat diet the healthiest way to eat?**

1. Walter C. Willet, Meir J. Stampfer, "Rebuild the food pyramid," *Scientific American,* January 2003, pp. 64–71.
2. Walter C. Willet, F. B. Hu, "Optimal diets for prevention of coronary heart disease," *Journal of the American Medical Association,* v. 288, November 27, 2002, pp. 2569–2578.

**Question #96: Are low-carb diets effective for weight loss?**

1. G. D. Foster, H. R. Wyatt, et al., "A randomized trial of a low-carbohydrate diet for obesity," *New England Journal of Medicine,* v. 348, May 2003, pp. 2082–2090.
2. F. F. Samaha, N. Igbal, et al., "A low-carbohydrate as compared with a low-fat diet in severe obesity," *New England Journal of Medicine,* v. 348, May 2003, pp. 2074–2081.
3. J. H. Ware, "Interpreting incomplete data in studies of diet and weight loss," *New England Journal of Medicine,* v. 348, May 2003, pp. 2236–2137.

**Question #97: Why do low-carb diets seem to be effective in the short run?**

Bonnie Brehm, Randy Seeley, et al., "A randomized trial comparing a very low carbohydrate diet and a calorie-restricted low fat diet on body weight and cardiovascular risk factors in healthy women," *Journal of Clinical Endocrinology and Metabolism,* v. 88, April 2003, pp. 1617–1623.

**Question #98: Do I need more protein if I exercise?**

1. Janet W. Rankin, "Role of protein in exercise," *Clinical Sports Medicine,* v. 18, July 1999, pp. 499–511.
2. R. A. Fielding, "What are the dietary protein requirements of physically active individuals? New evidence on the effects of exercise on protein utilization during post-exercise recovery," *Nutrition in Clinical Care,* v. 5, July 1, 2002, pp. 191–196.

**Question #99: Could fast food really be addictive?**

Jiali Wang, Silvana Obici, Kimyata Morgan, et al., "Overfeeding rapidly induces leptin and insulin resistance," *Diabetes,* v. 50, 2001, pp. 2786–2791.

**Question #100: Can fiber help me lose weight?**

1. N. C. Howarth, E. Saltzman, Susan Roberts, "Dietary fiber and weight regulation," *Nutrition Review,* v. 59, May 2001, pp. 129–139.
2. Susan B. Roberts, Megan A. McCrory, Edward Saltzman, "The influence of dietary composition on energy intake and body weight," *Journal of the American College of Nutrition,* v. 21, April 2002, pp. 141S–142S.

**Question #101: Will artificial sweeteners help me lose weight?**

A. Raben, T. Vasilaras, et al., "Sucrose compared with artificial sweeteners: Different effects on ad libitum food intake and body weight after 10 wk of supplementation in overweight subjects," *American Journal of Clinical Nutrition,* v. 76, October 2002, pp. 721–729.

**Question #104: Will drinking lots of water help me lose weight?**

Barbara Rolls et al., "Water incorporated into a food but not served with a food decreases energy intake in lean women," *American Journal of Clinical Nutrition,* v. 70, October 1999, pp. 448–455.

**Question #105: How much water should I drink when I work out?**

T. D. Hew, J. N. Chorley, et al., "The incidence, risk factors, and clinical manifestations of hyponatremia in marathon runners," *Clinical Journal of Sports Medicine,* v. 13, January 2003, pp. 41–47.

**Question #109: Will Slim Fast and other "meal-replacement" shakes really help me lose weight?**

S. B. Heymsfield, C. A. van Mierlo, et al., "Weight management using a meal replacement strategy: Meta and pooling analysis from six studies," *International Journal of Obesity and Related Metabolic Disorders,* v. 27, May 2003, pp. 537–549.

**Question #114: How much exercise do I really need?**

1. *Dietary Reference Intakes for Energy, Carbohydrate, Fiber, Fat, Fatty Acids, Cholesterol, Protein, and Amino Acids (Macronutrients)* (Washington, D.C.: The National Academies Press, 2002), pp. 697–736.
2. *Physical Activity and Health, A Report of the Surgeon General* (Washington, D.C.: U.S. Department of Health and Human Services, 1996).
3. Steven Blair et al., "Physical fitness and activity as separate heart disease risk factors: a meta-analysis," *Medicine & Science in Sports & Exercise,* v. 33, May 2001, pp. 762–764.

**Question #115: Do I have to work out for 30 consecutive minutes or are shorter workouts just as effective?**

W. D. Schmidt, C. J. Biwer, et al., "Effects of long versus short bout exercise on fitness and weight loss in overweight females," *Journal of the American College of Nutrition,* v. 20, October 2001, pp. 494–501.

**Question #116: Can I get in shape by doing gardening, housework, and other so-called "lifestyle activities"?**

J. P. Koplan, C. J. Caspersen, et al., "Physical activity, physical fitness, and health: Time to act," *Journal of the American Medical Association,* v. 262, November 3, 1989, p. 2437.

**Question #119: What exactly is the *target zone*?**

Edward T. Howley, "Type of activity: Resistance, aerobic and leisure versus occupational physical activity," *Medicine & Science in Sports & Exercise,* v. 33 (Supplement), 2001, pp. S364–S369.

**Question #135: Which delivers a better workout, an upright stationary cycle or a recumbent stationary cycle?**

Marsha A. Pauly, "A comparison of the submaximal and maximal responses to upright versus semi-recumbent cycling in females," graduate thesis, University of Wisconsin–La Crosse, December 1999.

**Question #136: Is inline skating a good fitness activity?**

A. C. Synder, K. P. O'Hagan, et al., "Physiological responses to in-line skating compared to treadmill running," *International Journal of Sports Medicine,* v. 14, January 1993, pp. 38–42.

**Question #137: How did the marathon distance come to be 26.2 miles?**

1. Hal Higdon, *Marathon: The Ultimate Training Guide* (Emmaus, Pa.: Rodale Press, 1999), pp. 5–8.
2. David E. Martin, Roger W. H. Gynn, *The Olympic Marathon: The History and Drama of Sport's Most Challenging Event* (Champaign, Ill.: Human Kinetics, 2000), pp. 5–6 and 57–58.

**Question #145: Can I strengthen and tone my muscles with rubber exercise bands or tubes?**

K. W. Jones, et al., "Predicting forces applied by Thera-Band during resistive exercises," *Journal of Orthopaedic & Sports Physical Therapy,* v. 27, 1998, p. 65.

**Question #146: How many days a week should I lift weights?**

Edward T. Howley, "Type of activity: Resistance, aerobic and leisure versus occupational physical activity," *Medicine & Science in Sports & Exercise,* v. 33 (Supplement), 2001, pp. S364–S369.

**Question #147: Is there any benefit to lifting weights just once a week if that's all the time I have?**

J. R. McLester, P. Bishop, M. Guilliams, "Comparison of 1 and 3 days per week of equal volume resistance training in experienced subjects," *Medicine & Science in Sports & Exercise,* v. 31 (Supplement), 1999, p. S117.

**Question #150: Is one set of strength-training exercises as effective as three?**

1. S. P. Messier, M. E. Dill, "Alterations in strength and maximal

oxygen uptake consequent to Nautilus circuit weight training," *Research Quarterly for Exercise and Sport,* v. 56, 1985, pp. 345–351.

2. L. J. Silvester, C. Stiggins, et al., "Effect of variable resistance and free-weight training programs on strength and vertical jump," *National Strength and Conditioning Association Journal,* v. 3, 1981–1982, pp. 30–33.

**Question #158: I've heard the Super Slow method of weight training is more effective than lifting weights at a normal speed. Is this true?**

1. Wayne Westcott et al., "Effects of regular and slow speed resistance training on muscle strength," *Journal of Sports Medicine and Physical Fitness,* v. 41, June 2001, pp. 154–158.

2. G. R. Hunter, D. Seelhorst, S. Snyder, "Comparison of metabolic and heart rate responses to Super Slow vs. traditional resistance training," *Journal of Strength and Conditioning Research,* v. 1, February 2003, pp. 76–81.

**Question #166: Is the crunch the best way to work your abs?**

"New study puts the crunch on ineffective ab exercises," *ACE Fitness Matters,* v. 7, May–June 2001, pp. 21–23.

**Question #170: Should I wear a weight belt when pumping iron?**

R. J. Giorcelli, R. E. Hughes, "The effect of wearing a back belt on spine kinematics during asymmetric lifting of large and small boxes," *Spine,* v. 26, August 15, 2001, pp. 1794–1798.

**Question #171: Is it safe for kids to lift weights?**

"Strength training by children and adolescents," *Pediatrics,* v. 107, June 2001, pp. 1470–1472.

**Question #182: Can electronic muscle stimulation belts really tone my abs?**

John Porcari, "Electrical muscle stimulations: Highly charged workout or hair-raising experience?" *ACE Fitness Matters,* v. 6, May–June 2000, pp. 11–13.

**Question #185: How accurate are pedometers?**

1. Patrick Schneider et al., "Pedometer measures of free-living physical activity: Comparison of 13 models," *Medicine & Science in*

*Sports & Exercise,* v. 36, February 2004, pp. 331–335.

2. S. E. Crouter et al., "Validity of 10 electronic pedometers for measuring steps, distance, and energy cost," *Medicine & Science in Sports & Exercise,* v. 35, August 2003, pp. 1455–1460.

**Question #192: Do exercisers get sick less often than people who don't work out?**

1. David C. Nieman, Bente K. Pedersen, "Exercise and immune function: Recent developments," *Sports Medicine,* v. 27, February 1999, pp. 73–80.

2. David C. Nieman, "Is infection risk linked to exercise workload?" *Medicine & Science in Sports & Exercise,* v. 32, July 2000, pp. S406–S411.

**Question #193: Am I more likely to get sick after a killer workout than a more moderate one?**

1. David C. Nieman, Bente K. Pedersen, "Exercise and immune function: Recent developments," *Sports Medicine,* v. 27, February 1999, pp. 73–80.

2. David C. Nieman, "Is infection risk linked to exercise workload?" *Medicine & Science in Sports & Exercise,* v. 32, July 2000, pp. S406–S411.

**Question #199: What fitness activity has the highest injury rate?**

Ralph K. Requa, L. Nicole DeAvilla, James G. Garrick, "Injuries in recreational adult fitness activities," *American Journal of Sports Medicine,* v. 21, 1993, pp. 461–467.

**Question #201: Will I sleep better if I exercise?**

1. Shawn Youngstedt, Patrick J. O'Connor, Rod K. Dishman, "The effects of acute exercise on sleep: A quantitative synthesis," *Sleep,* v. 20, March 1997, pp. 203–214.

2. Shawn Youngstedt, Michael L. Perlis, et al., "No association of sleep with total daily physical activity in normal sleepers," *Physiology & Behavior,* v. 78, March 2003, pp. 395–401.

**Question #202: Will a hard workout close to bedtime keep me awake?**

Shawn Youngstedt, Daniel Kripke, and Jeffrey Elliott, "Is sleep disturbed by vigorous late-night exercise?" *Medicine & Science in Sports & Exercise,* v. 31, June 1999, pp. 864–869.

### Question #203: If I don't get enough sleep, will my workouts suffer?

1. G. Himashree, P. K. Banerjee, et al., "Sleep and performance — recent trends," *Indian Journal of Physiology and Pharmacology,* v. 46, January 2002, pp. 6–24.
2. J. J. Pilcher, A. I. Huffcutt, "Effects of sleep deprivation on performance: A meta-analysis," *Sleep,* v. 19, May 1996, pp. 318–326.
3. T. VanHelder, M. W. Radomski, "Sleep deprivation and the effect on exercise performance," *Sports Medicine,* v. 7, April 1989, pp. 235–247.

### Question #208: Can exercise help treat clinical depression?

Alisha L. Brosse, Erin S. Sheets, et al., "Exercise and the treatment of clinical depression in adults: Recent findings and future directions," *Sports Medicine,* v. 32, pp. 741–760.

### Question #211: I keep hearing about Syndrome X and the health problems related to it. What exactly is this condition?

Y. W. Park, S. Zhu, et al., "The metabolic syndrome: prevalence and associated risk factor findings in the U.S. population from the third National Health and Nutrition Examination Survey, 1988–1994," *Archive of Internal Medicine,* v. 163, February 24, 2003, pp. 395–397.

### Question #212: If I'm overweight, am I at greater risk for developing cancer?

Eugenia Calle, Carmen Rodgriguez, "Overweight, obesity, and mortality from cancer in a prospectively studied cohort of U.S. adults," *New England Journal of Medicine,* v. 348, April 24, 2003, pp. 1625–1638.

### Question #217: Will stretching reduce my risk of injury?

1. R. D. Herbert, M. Gabriel, "Effects of stretching before and after exercising on muscle soreness and risk of injury: systematic review," *British Medical Journal,* v. 325, August 31, 2002, p. 468.
2. David A. Lally, "Stretching and injury in distance runners," *Medicine & Science in Sports & Exercise,* v. 26 (Supplement), 1994, p. S437.

### Question #219: How long should I hold a stretch?

W. D. Bandy, J. M. Irion, M. Briggler, "The effect of static stretch and dynamic range of motion training on the flexibility of the hamstring muscles," *Journal of Orthopaedic and Sports Physical Therapy,* v. 27, April 1998, pp. 295–300.

**Question #220: I tend to skimp on my stretching because it's painful. Is there an alternative method I can try?**

Phil Wharton, Jim Wharton, *The Whartons' Stretch Book* (New York: Times Books, 1996).

**Question #221: My trainer recommended PNF stretching. How is this different from regular stretching?**

"American College of Sports Medicine position stand," *Medicine & Science in Sports & Exercise,* v. 30, June 1998, pp. 975–991.

**Question #223: Can yoga help me lose weight?**

T. Schmidt, A. Wijga, et al., "Changes in cardiovascular risk factors and hormones during a comprehensive residential three month kriya yoga training and vegetarian nutrition," *Acta Physiologica Scandinavica Supplement,* v. 640, 1997, pp. 158–162.

**Question #231: Is it safe to exercise when I'm pregnant?**

1. American College of Obstetricians and Gynecologists, *Exercise During Pregnancy and the Postpartum Period.* Technical Bulletin No. 189 (Washington, D.C.: ACOG, 1994).
2. "ACOG Committee opinion. Number 267, January 2002: Exercise during pregnancy and the postpartum period," *Obstetrics and Gynecology,* v. 99, January 2002, pp. 171–173.
3. James F. Clapp III, *Exercising Through Your Pregnancy* (Champaign, Ill.: Human Kinetics, 1998), pp. 3–15.
4. James F. Clapp III, "Exercise during pregnancy: A clinical update," *Clinical Sports Medicine,* v. 19, April 2000, pp. 273–286.

**Question #232: If I exercise while I'm pregnant, will I have an easier labor?**

James F. Clapp III, *Exercising Through Your Pregnancy* (Champaign, Ill.: Human Kinetics, 1998), pp. 93–95.

**Question #233: Will I gain less weight during pregnancy if I exercise?**

1. James F. Clapp III, *Exercising Through Your Pregnancy* (Champaign, Ill.: Human Kinetics, 1998), pp. 82–83.

2. James F. Clapp III, "Exercise during pregnancy: A clinical up-date," *Clinical Sports Medicine,* v. 19, April 2000, pp. 273–286.

### Question #234: Will I ever be as fit after pregnancy as I was before?

1. James F. Clapp III, Eleanor Capeless, "The VO2 max of recre-ational athletes before and after pregnancy," *Medicine & Science in Sports & Exercise,* v. 23, October 1991, pp. 1128–1133.
2. Helene Elliott, "Pregnant pause," *Los Angeles Times,* April 10, 2003, p. D1.

### Question #235: Will working out affect how much breast milk I pro-duce or what it tastes like to my baby?

1. Kathryn G. Dewey, C. A. Lovelady, et al., "A randomized study of the effects of aerobic exercise by lactating women on breast-milk volume and composition," *New England Journal of Medi-cine,* v. 330, February 17, 1994, pp. 449–453.
2. James F. Clapp III, *Exercising Through Your Pregnancy* (Cham-paign, Ill.: Human Kinetics, 1998), pp. 72–75.

### Question #237: What's the best way to lose weight after pregnancy?

1. Kathryn G. Dewey, "Effects of maternal caloric restriction and exercise during lactation," *Journal of Nutrition,* v. 128, February 1998, pp. 386S–389S.
2. Megan A. McCrory, Laurie A. Nommsen-Rivers, et al., "Ran-domized trial of the short-term effects of dieting compared with dieting plus aerobic exercise on lactation performance," *Ameri-can Journal of Clinical Nutrition,* v. 69, May 1999, pp. 959–967.

### Question #238: Will I gain weight permanently after having a baby?

Dawnine Enette Larson-Meyer, "Effect of postpartum exercise on mothers and their offspring: A review of the literature," *Obesity Research,* v. 10, August 2002, pp. 841–853.

# Index

Page numbers in *italics* refer to illustrations.

# About the Authors

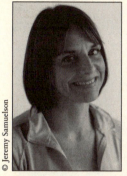

© Jeremy Samuelson

**Liz Neporent** holds a master's degree in exercise physiology and is certified by the American College of Sports Medicine, the National Strength and Conditioning Association, and the American Council on Exercise, for which she serves on the board of directors. As the Fit by Friday columnist for iVillage.com, the leading Internet site for women's issues, Liz fields weekly fitness and weight-loss questions. She is also the author of numerous books, including *Fitness Walking for Dummies, The Ultimate Body: 10 Perfect Workouts for Women,* and, with Suzanne Schlosberg, *Fitness for Dummies* and *Weight Training for Dummies*. In addition to being a writer, Liz is a sought-after personal trainer and fitness consultant. When she's not busy spreading the word about health and fitness, she is out with her husband, Jay Shafran, running, rock climbing, hiking, or poring over the latest science journals.

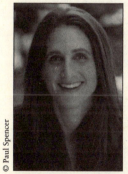

© Paul Spencer

**Suzanne Schlosberg** balances a dual career as a fitness writer and a humorist. A contributing editor to *Shape,* Suzanne writes the magazine's Weight Loss Q&A and Fitness Q&A columns. She is the author of *The Ultimate Workout Log,* now in its third edition, and *Fitness for Travelers,* and she is the coauthor, with Liz Neporent, of *Fitness for Dummies* and *Weight Training for Dummies*. A competitive cyclist and avid weightlifter, Suzanne is the women's record holder in the Great American Sack Race, a quadrennial event held in Yerington, Nevada, in which competitors run 5 miles while carrying a 50-pound sack of chicken feed. Suzanne's victory is chronicled in *Sand in My Bra: Funny Women Write from the Road*. Her most recent book is *The Curse of the Singles Table: A True Story of 1001 Nights Without Sex*. Suzanne lives in Bend, Oregon, with her husband, Paul Spencer, and can be reached at SuzanneSchlosberg.com.